The Arthritis Helpbook

ADDISON-WESLEY PUBLISHING COMPANY

Reading, Massachusetts • Menlo Park, California • New York • Don Mills, Ontario Wokingham, England • Amsterdam • Bonn • Sydney • Singapore • Tokyo • Madrid San Juan • Paris • Seoul • Milan • Mexico City • Taipei

▼ ▼ ▼ ▼ ▼ ▼ ▼ ▼ ▼ ▼

The Arthritis Helpbook

A Tested Self-Management Program for Coping with Arthritis and Fibromyalgia

FOURTH EDITION

Kate Lorig, R.N., Dr. P.H.
Director, Patient Education Research
Stanford Arthritis Center

James F. Fries, M.D.
Professor of Medicine
Stanford University School of Medicine

CONTRIBUTORS

Maureen R. Gecht, O.T.R./L., M.P.H., Occupational Therapist

Marian Minor, R.P.T., Ph.D., Physical Therapist

Diana D. Laurent, M.P.H., Health Educator

Virginia M. González, M.P.H., Health Educator

Nancy L. Brannigan, Illustrator

Many of the designations used by manufacturers and sellers to distinguish their products are claimed as trademarks. Where those designations appear in this book and Addison-Wesley was aware of a trademark claim, the designations have been printed in initial capital letters (e.g., Tylenol, Water-Pik). Aspirin is a registered trademark in Canada.

This book is not meant to replace medical care. If you are under the care of a doctor and other health professionals, follow their advice first. Read medicine labels fully because instructions may vary from year to year. If any problem persists beyond a reasonable time, see a doctor.

Library of Congress Cataloging-in-Publication Data
Lorig, Kate.
    The arthritis helpbook : a tested self-management program for coping with arthritis and fibromyalgia / Kate Lorig, James F. Fries; contributors, Maureen R. Gecht ... [et al.]. — 4th ed.
      p.   cm.
    Includes bibliographical references and index.
    ISBN 0-201-40963-1
    1. Arthritis — Popular works.   2. Fibromyalgia — Popular works.
I. Fries, James F.   II. Title.
RC933.L628   1995
616.7′22 — dc20   94-48208
          CIP

Cover design by Suzanne Heiser
Text design by Joyce C. Weston
Set in 11 1/2-point Minion by Douglas & Gayle, Ltd., Indianapolis, Indiana

8 9 10 11 12 13-CRS-0100999897
Eigth printing, April 1997

Addison-Wesley books are available at special discounts for bulk purchases. For more information about how to make such purchases, please contact the publisher.

In the U.S.:	In Canada:
Corporate, Government, and	Special Markets Department
Special Sales Department	Addison-Wesley Publishing Company
Addison-Wesley Publishing Company	26 Prince Andrew Place
1 Jacob Way	Don Mills, Ontario M3C 2T8
Reading, MA 01867	(800) 387-8028
(800) 238-9682	

To our more than 2,000 class leaders
and over 150,000
Arthritis Self-Help class participants
around the world

▼ ▼ ▼ ▼ ▼ ▼ ▼

Contents

▼ ▼ ▼ ▼ ▼ ▼ ▼

Acknowledgments

We would like especially to thank the Stanford Arthritis Center folks: Pat Spitz, Gene Fauro Pratt, Audrey Schomer, R. Guy Kraines, Jim Standish, Alison Harlow, Cathy Williams, Dr. Dennis McShane, Dr. Jeffrey Brown, Dr. Cody Wasner, Dr. Paul Feigenbaum, Dr. Halsted Holman, Dr. Andrei Calin, Dr. Melvin Britton, Dr. Tom Okarma, Dr. William Lages, Dr. David Schurman, Dr. Linda Lee, Dr. Robert Marcus, Patricia Schweikert, Steve Wilson, Vicky Brey, Catherine Regan, and Larissa Ortiz. A special thanks goes to Connie Hartnett, who has given invaluable support over the years.

The Stanford Midpeninsula Health Clinic people: Dr. Joseph Hopkins, Judy Staples, Jeanne Ewy, Virginia de Lemos, Sally Semans, and Debbie Stinchfield.

The University of California at Berkeley Health Education Faculty: Dr. Robert Miller, Dr. Andrew Fisher, Dr. William Griffiths, Dr. Meredith Minkler, Dr. Carol D'Onofrio, and Dr. John Ratcliffe.

Significant others: Dr. Robert Swezey, John Staples, Donna Holsten, Dr. Lawrence Green, Dr. Sarah Archer, Janice Pigg, Dr. Floyd Pennington, Dr. Stan Shoor, Dr. Peter Wood, Melinda Seeger, Dr. Larry Bradley, Michele Boutaugh, Roseanne Glick, Dr. Ann O'Leary, Dr. B. Shapiro, Gail Schreiber, and Dr. F. Keefe. A special thanks to our Canadian First Nations leaders and class participants.

Many people have kindly agreed to review sections of this edition. Their comments have made us rethink and rewrite. To all of you, many thanks.

In addition, many people in various countries have written us and reveiwed and added to our materials.

AUSTRALIA
Pauline Brooks, Physiotherapist M.C.S.P., Adelaide
Jenny Davidson, R.N., Melbourne
Valerie Sayce, B.A., D.I.P., Physiotherapist, Melbourne
Peter Brooks, M.D., F.R.A.C.P., Sydney

CANADA
Paul Adams, M.S.W., Vancouver
Sally Frost, R.P.T., Vancouver
Sherry Lynch, B.S.W., Vancouver
Patrick McGowan, M.S.W., Vancouver
Greg Taylor, B.S.W., Vancouver

NEW ZEALAND
Pam Antill, Auckland
Chree Barker, Auckland
Gwynneth Carter, Physiotherapist, Wellington
Marie Gilles, Wellington
Nerida Miller, Napier

UNITED STATES
Barbara F. Banwell, P.T., Ann Arbor
Bruce F. Campbell, Ph.D., Palo Alto
Victoria Gall, R.P.T., M.Ed., Boston
Kathleen M. Haralson, P.T., St. Louis
Linda Lee, M.D., Stanford
Robert Marcus, M.D., Stanford
Carolee Moncur, P.T., Ph.D., Salt Lake City
Linda G. Price, M.A., Columbia

GREAT BRITAIN
Ann Rodriguez
Margaret A. Byron, M.D., F.R.C.P.

SOUTH AFRICA
Gil Brown

Finally, thanks to the many people coping with arthritis who have posed for the photos.

▼ ▼ ▼ ▼ ▼ ▼ ▼

Preface

*B*EFORE we start, we would like to say a little about how this book came to be written and what we have learned in the process.

In 1979 the Stanford Arthritis Center began giving lessons to people with arthritis. (From the very beginning our class members told us that they did not want to be called patients.) The classes were taught by forty people from our community who had arthritis or who were interested in arthritis. With a few exceptions, the teachers were not health professionals. The Arthritis Center staff worked with the teachers, and the lay teachers led the classes.

Our arthritis education classes use the same principles we presented earlier in *Take Care of Yourself, Taking Care of Your Child, Arthritis,* and, most recently, *Living Well.* They have benefited greatly from the many thousands of encouraging letters and helpful suggestions we have received. In these classes we are not concerned solely with improving knowledge. We also seek to help people with arthritis change their activities and abilities, decrease their pain, and, most important, develop more confidence in themselves as caretakers for their bodies.

In our classes we emphasize three concepts:

1. Each person with arthritis is different. There is no one treatment that is right for everyone.
2. There are a number of things people can do to feel better. These things will not cure most kinds of arthritis, but they will help to relieve pain, maintain or increase mobility, and prevent deformity.
3. With knowledge, each individual is the best judge of which self-management techniques are best for him or her.

Therefore, this book was developed to give details about a variety of self-management treatments. We felt that it was not enough just to know that you should exercise. Instead, you must know about particular exercises, types of exercise, when to exercise, and how much to exercise. You need to understand the relationship between exercise and pain. The same considerations hold for what you need to know about relaxation, nutrition, problem solving, and all other self-management techniques. In *Arthritis: A Take Care of Yourself Health Guide,* Jim Fries provided all the factual knowledge about arthritis. In this companion volume he and Kate Lorig try to help you use the information. This is a how-to-do-it book that has been developed with the help of many people very much like you.

When our class members first used this book they liked it but were quick to point out its faults: a neck exercise that caused too much pain, a nutrition section that was unclear, omission of a section on sleep disturbances, and so forth. Taking these suggestions we have added, revised, clarified, reused, re-revised in a continuing cycle that has resulted in this present edition.

While only seven names appear on the title page as authors and contributors, this book was really written and guided by you, people with arthritis. As of late 1994, more than 150,000 people have attended the classes we developed and used this book. This small program which started at Stanford University has spread to Australia, New Zealand, Canada, South Africa, Great Britain, Denmark, Iceland, Finland, the Czech Republic, and Lithuania. From all our friends around the world we have gained insights that we hope will be helpful to you.

All these people helped us in other ways, too. We have been carefully studying the effect of our classes on the way people get along with their arthritis, and our class members have served as the subjects for these studies. In effect, we "drew straws" to see which of the subjects on the waiting list would attend the next set of classes and which would have to wait four months. Then we compared how the people who went to the classes did with how the people on the waiting list did. Data from long questionnaires went into the computer, and after elaborate analyses we found what we had suspected all along.

People who become good arthritis self-managers have less pain and are more active than those people who feel there is nothing they can do for themselves. These were among the first controlled studies that have ever been done relating education programs in arthritis to outcomes, and they are very encouraging. The bottom line is that arthritis self-managers feel better! We would like to help you become an arthritis self-manager.

Now a few words of caution. First, you did not get stiff, painful joints overnight. Therefore, relief will not come quickly. Self-management is in no way a quick cure; it is a way of life to be practiced every day for the rest of your life. However, it is never too late to start. Our oldest self-manager was 100 when she first came to class.

Second, not everything works for everyone. Experiment, but give each activity two weeks to a month for first results. Don't give up too soon. If one thing does not work for you, try another.

This book is not meant to replace medical care. Rather, it is a supplement to that care. Most doctors do not have or do not take the time to explain exercises or pain-management techniques in enough detail to help you very much. Therefore, we are hopeful that this book will assist both you and your physician. All of the advice and activities that we describe have been reviewed by many, many doctors, physical therapists, occupational therapists, nutritionists, and nurses, including the entire staff of the Stanford Arthritis Center. They represent a sound program essentially the same as that recommended by most health authorities today. If you have particular questions please talk them over with your doctor.

Finally, if you are reading this book after the year 2005, the information is probably somewhat out of date. Things do change. Check with your bookseller or library to find out if there is a more recent edition of this *Helpbook* available.

We would like you to feel that you are part of our cast of thousands. If you have comments or suggestions please send them to us by writing:

Stanford Arthritis Center
1000 Welch Road, Suite 204
Palo Alto, CA 94304
U.S.A.

Your suggestions will be reviewed and considered for our next edition. To all of you who helped in the past and whom we couldn't name, many thanks, and to those of you who are just joining, a hearty welcome.

Stanford, California   K. L.
March 1995   J. F. F.

▼ ▼ ▼ ▼ ▼ ▼ ▼ ▼ ▼ ▼ ▼

PART ONE

Understanding Those Aches and Pains

1. Arthritis: What Is It?

ARTHRITIS. The very word evokes a specter of fear and pain. People think of getting old, being unable to get around, and of becoming more dependent upon others. More so than with any other disease, the term *arthritis* carries with it a sense of hopelessness and futility. But the very opposite should be true. All arthritis can be helped.

In order to understand how to work with your arthritis, it is necessary to know a little about it. In fact, arthritis is not just a single disease. There are over 120 kinds of arthritis, all of which have something to do with one or more joints in the body. Even the word *arthritis* is misleading. The *arth*-part comes from the Greek word meaning "joint," while *-itis* means "inflammation or infection." Thus, the word *arthritis* means "inflammation of the joint." The problem is that in many kinds of arthritis, the joint is not inflamed. A better description might be "problems with the joint."

The next step is to understand what a joint looks like and what the various parts do.

A joint is a meeting of two bones for the purpose of allowing movement. It has the following six parts.

1. **Cartilage.** The end of each bone is covered with cartilage, a tough material that cushions and protects the ends of the bone. To get some idea of what cartilage is like, feel the middle of your nose or your ears. These are also made of cartilage. Cartilage in meat is gristle.
2. **Synovial membrane (synovial sac).** Around each joint is the synovial sac, which protects the joint and also secretes the synovial fluid, which oils the joint. In fact, this fluid has many times the lubricating power of oil. Synovial fluid is a little like egg white.
3. **Bursa.** A bursa is a small sac that is not part of the joint but is near the joint. It contains a fluid that lubricates the movement of muscles: muscle

Where Arthritis Attacks

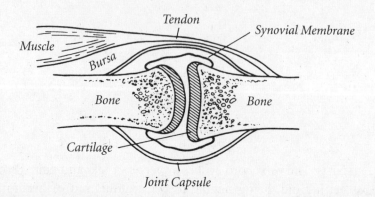

across muscle and muscle across bones. In some ways it is similar to the synovial sac.

4. **Muscle.** The muscles are elastic tissues that, by becoming shorter and longer, move the bones and thus move you.
5. **Tendon.** The tendons are fibrous cords that attach the muscles to the bones. You can feel them on the back of your hand or in the back of your knee.
6. **Ligament.** The ligaments are much shorter fibrous cords that attach bone to bone and make up the joint capsules.

When someone says, "I have arthritis," it means that something is wrong with one or more of these parts. For example, when the synovial membrane becomes inflamed, this is true arthritis. That is, the joint is inflamed. However, if the muscle becomes stretched from overexercise or is injured, this is not arthritis. The joint itself is not affected.

In each major kind of arthritis, a different joint tissue is involved. In *rheumatoid arthritis,* the problem is chiefly *synovitis,* that is, an inflammation of the synovial membrane. This inflammation must be reduced with medication in addition to your self-management program. In *ankylosing spondylitis,* the problem is an *enthesopathy,* an inflammation where the ligaments attach to the bone. This inflammation also needs to be suppressed by medication, and the affected joints need to be regularly and vigorously stretched. In *osteoarthritis,* the problem is a breakdown of the joint cartilage, but it is helped by exercise and proper use of your joints. In *gout,* the problem is crystals that form in the joint space and cause inflammation and pain. Each kind of arthritis is different, and different treatment is needed.

Here is a quick overview of the three most common types of arthritis.

TYPES OF ARTHRITIS

PATHOLOGY	RHEUMATOID ARTHRITIS	OSTEOARTHRITIS	FIBROMYALGIA
What happens	Inflammation of synovial membrane, bone destruction, damage to ligaments, tendons, cartilage, joint capsule.	Cartilage degeneration; bone regeneration (growth) may result in bone spurs.	Unknown. Accompanied by sleep disturbance and prolonged muscle contraction.
Joints affected	Symmetrical: wrists, knees, knuckles (both sides).	Hands, spine, knees, hips. May be one-sided.	Joints not affected. Certain tender points. Muscles, ligaments, tendons may be affected.
Features and symptoms	Swelling, redness, warmth, pain, tenderness, nodules, fatigue, stiffness, muscle aches, fever.	Localized pain, stiffness; bony knobs of end joints of fingers; usually not much swelling.	Overall aching, morning stiffness, fatigue. Sleep disturbance.
Long-term prognosis	Less aggressive with time; deformity can often be prevented.	Less pain for some, more pain and disability for others; few severely disabled.	Usually improves slowly over time. Pain and fatigue may be disabling in some, most are not disabled.
Age at onset	Adults in 20s to 50s, children approaching adolescence.	Age 45 to 90; most of us have some features with increasing age.	Age 30s to 50s.
Sex	75% female.	Males and females equally.	More frequently female.
Heredity	Familial tendency.	The form with knobby fingers can be familial.	Unknown at this time.
Tests	Rheumatoid factor (80%), blood tests, X-rays, examination of joint fluid.	X-rays.	Tender point exam, sometimes blood tests to exclude other conditions (thyroid tests, sedimentation rate).
Treatment	Reduce inflammation. Balanced exercise program, joint protection, weight control, relaxation, heat, sometimes medication and/or surgery.	Maintain activity level. Exercise, joint protection, weight control, relaxation, heat, sometimes medication and/or surgery.	Exercise, heat, relaxation, sometimes medication for pain and/or for enhancing sleep.

While there are over a hundred types of arthritis, we discuss in detail only the major types. If you are interested in knowing more about other types of arthritis, read *Arthritis: A Take Care of Yourself Health Guide,* by Dr. James F. Fries (Reading, Mass.: Addison-Wesley, 1995), or contact your local Arthritis Foundation or Arthritis Society for information.

REFERENCES

Arthritis Foundation. *Understanding Arthritis: What It Is, How It's Treated, How to Cope With It.* Ed. I. Kushner. New York: Scribner's, 1985.

Davidson, Paul. *Are You Sure It's Arthritis? A Guide to Soft-Tissue Rheumatism.* New York: New American Library, 1987.

Davidson, Paul. *Chronic Muscle Pain Syndrome.* New York: Villard, 1990.

Fries, James F. *Arthritis: A Take Care of Yourself Health Guide.* 4th ed. Reading, Mass.: Addison-Wesley, 1995.

2. Rheumatoid Arthritis: Inflamed Joints

RHEUMATOID arthritis (RA) is more than just arthritis. Indeed, many doctors call it "rheumatoid disease" to emphasize its widespread nature. The name is trying awkwardly to say the same thing; *rheum-* refers to the stiffness, body aching, and fatigue that often accompany rheumatoid arthritis. People with RA often describe feeling much as though they have a virus, with fatigue and aching in the muscles, except that, unlike with a usual viral illness, the condition may persist for months or even years.

About one half of one percent of the population has rheumatoid arthritis, about twenty million people around the world. Most of these people (about three quarters) are women. The condition usually appears in middle life, in the forties or fifties, although it can begin at any age. Rheumatoid arthritis in children is quite different. Rheumatoid arthritis has been medically identified for about two hundred years, although bone changes in the skeletons of some Mexican Indian groups suggest that the disease may have been around for thousands of years.

Since RA is so common, and because it can sometimes be severe, it is a major international health problem. It can result in difficulties with employment and problems with daily activities, and can put a severe stress on family relationships. In its most severe forms, and without good treatment, it can result in deformities of the joints. Fortunately, most people with RA do better than this, and most can lead normal lives. Fear of rheumatoid arthritis, sometimes greatly exaggerated, can be as harmful as the disease itself.

In RA, the synovial membrane lining in the joint becomes inflamed. We don't have a good explanation as to why this inflammation starts, but the cells in the membrane divide and grow, and inflammatory cells come into the joint. Because of the bulk of these inflammatory cells, the joint becomes swollen, and feels puffy or boggy to the touch. The increased blood flow that is a feature of the inflammation makes the joint warm. The cells release chemicals (called enzymes) into the joint space and the enzymes cause further irritation and pain. If the process continues for years, the enzymes may gradually digest the cartilage and bone of the joint, actually eating away parts of the bone.

This then is rheumatoid arthritis, a process in which inflammation of the joint membrane, over many years, can cause damage to the joint itself.

FEATURES

Swelling and pain in one or more joints, lasting at least six weeks, are required for a diagnosis of rheumatoid arthritis. Usually, both sides of the body are affected similarly, and the arthritis is said to be "symmetrical." Often there are slight differences between the two sides, usually the right side being slightly worse in right-handed people and vice versa. Occasionally the condition skips about in an erratic fashion. The wrists and knuckles are almost always involved. The knees and the joints of the ball of the foot are often involved as well, and any joint can be affected. Of the knuckles, those at the base of the fingers are most frequently painful, while the joints at the ends of the fingers are often normal.

Lumps, usually between the size of a pea and a mothball, may form beneath the skin. These *rheumatoid nodules* are most commonly located near the elbow at the place where you rest your arms on the table, but they can pop up anywhere. Each represents an inflammation of a small blood vessel. They come and go during the course of the illness and usually are not a big problem. They do tend to occur in people with the most severe kinds of RA. In rare cases, they become sore or infected, particularly if they are located around the ankle. Even more rarely, they form in the lungs or elsewhere in the body.

Laboratory tests can sometimes help a doctor recognize rheumatoid arthritis. The *rheumatoid factor* or *latex fixation* is the most commonly used blood test. Although this test may be negative in the first several months, it is eventually positive in about 80% of people with RA. The rheumatoid factor is actually an antibody to certain body proteins and can sometimes be found in individuals with other diseases. Some doctors think that it is a way the body fights the disease; others think that it may play a role in causing the joint damage.

The *sed rate* is another frequently used blood test. This test's full name is *erythrocyte sedimentation rate,* and the name sometimes is abbreviated ESR. The test doesn't help in diagnosis, but it does help tell the severity of the disease. A high sed rate (over 30 or so) suggests that the disease is quite active. The joint fluid is sometimes examined in rheumatoid arthritis in order to look at the inflammatory cells or to make sure that the joint is not infected with bacteria.

X-rays are not very helpful in the initial diagnosis of rheumatoid arthritis. It is unusual for changes to be seen in the bones or cartilage in the first few months of the disease, even when it is most severe. X-rays can help the doctor determine if damage to the bones or cartilage has occurred as the disease progresses. Some doctors like to get baseline X-rays to compare with later X-rays. Simple hand X-rays probably should be done in the first year of disease and every two or three years thereafter.

Most people with RA notice problems in parts of their bodies other than the joints themselves. Usually, there are general problems such as muscle aches, fatigue, muscle stiffness (particularly in the morning), and even a low fever. Morning stiffness is often considered a hallmark of RA and is sometimes termed the *gel phenomenon*. After a rest period or even after just sitting motionless for a few minutes, the whole body feels stiff and is difficult to move. After a period of loosening up, motion becomes easier and less painful. People often have problems with fluid accumulation, particularly around the ankles. Occasionally, the rheumatoid disease may attack other body tissues, including the whites of the eyes, the nerves, the small arteries, and the lungs. Anemia (low red-blood-cell count) is quite common, although it is seldom severe enough to need any treatment. Some patients will develop *Sjögren's disease,* or sicca syndrome, in which the tear fluids and the saliva dry up, causing dry eyes and dry mouth. This happens because the lacrimal (tear) glands and the salivary glands become involved in the rheumatoid process.

There can be unusual features that are due to the inflammation of the joint membrane. A *Baker's cyst* can form behind the knees and may feel like a tumor. It is just the synovial sac full of fluid, but it can extend down into the back of the calf and may cause pain. Or, the fluid in the joint can become infected and require immediate treatment. Suspect this if a single joint, usually a knee, becomes suddenly and severely worse.

Rheumatoid arthritis is one of the most complicated and mysterious diseases known. It is a challenge to patient and physician alike. Fortunately, the course of RA can be dramatically changed in most individuals. More so than with any other form of arthritis, if you have RA you need to develop an effective partnership with your doctor, as discussed in Chapter 19.

PROGNOSIS (WHAT WILL HAPPEN IN THE FUTURE)

Rheumatoid arthritis is the condition that most people think of when they hear the word *arthritis*. An image that comes to mind is of a person in a wheelchair, with swollen knees and twisted hands. True, most such people have rheumatoid arthritis. On balance, rheumatoid arthritis is the most destructive kind of arthritis known. Erosion of the bone itself, rupture of tendons, and slippage of the joints can result in crippling. But most people with rheumatoid arthritis do very much better than this. Many of the serious problems can be prevented by good, early treatment.

Often it is hard for persons with RA and their relatives to appreciate that inflammation in even the worst forms of rheumatoid arthritis tends to lessen with time. The arthritis usually becomes less aggressive. The inflammation (synovitis) is less active and the fatigue and stiffness decrease. New joints are less likely to become involved after several years of disease. But even though the disease is less violent, any destruction of bones and ligaments that occurred in earlier years will persist. Thus, deformities usually will not improve, even though no new damage is occurring. Hence, it is important to treat the disease correctly in the early years so that the joints will work well after the disease activity subsides.

TREATMENT

Treatment programs for RA are often complicated and can be confusing. In this section we give the broad outlines for sound management. But you need to work out with your doctor the combination of measures that is best for you. It has been said that the person who has himself for a doctor has a fool for a patient. In many areas of medicine, and for some kinds of arthritis, this is not true—you can do just as well looking out for yourself. But with rheumatoid arthritis you do need a doctor. Indeed, with rheumatoid arthritis, we strongly believe that you should be seen early in the course of the disease by a specialist in arthritis, a rheumatologist. In this way, the critical early treatment can begin at the right time. Only rheumatologists are familiar with the latest and most effective RA treatments.

First, some common sense. Your RA may be with you, on and off, for months or years. The best treatments are those that will help you maintain a life that is as nearly normal as possible. Often the worst treatments are those that offer immediate relief. They may allow joint damage to progress or may cause delayed side effects that ultimately make you feel worse. So you must develop some patience with the disease and with its management. You have to adjust your thinking to operate in the same slow time scale that the disease uses. You and your doctor will want to be anticipating problems before they occur so that they may be avoided. The adjustment to a long-term illness, with the necessity to plan treatment programs that may take months to get results, is a difficult psychological task. This adjustment will be one of your hardest jobs in battling your arthritis.

Synovitis is the underlying problem. The inflammation of the joint membrane releases enzymes that very slowly damage the joint structures. Good treatment reduces this inflammation and stops the damage. Painkillers can increase comfort but do not decrease the arthritis. In fact, pain per se helps to protect the joints by discouraging too much use. Therefore, in RA it is important to treat pain by treating the inflammation that causes the pain. By and large, pain relievers such as codeine, Percodan, Darvon, or Demerol must be avoided. (To learn more, read Chapter 20.)

The proper balance between rest and exercise is hard to understand. Rest reduces the inflammation, and this is good. But rest also lets joints get stiff and muscles get weak. With too much rest, tendons become less strong and bones get softer. Obviously, this is bad. So moderation is the basic principle. It may help you to know that your body usually gives you the right signals about what to do and what not to do. If it hurts too much, don't do it. If you don't seem to have much problem with an activity, go ahead. As a general rule, if you continue to have exercise-caused pain for more than two hours after exercising, you have done too much.

A particularly painful joint may require a splint to help it rest. Still, you will want to exercise the joint by stretching it gently in different directions to keep it from getting stiff. You will not want to use a splint for too long, or you may want to use it just at night. As the joint gets better, you will want to begin using the joint, gently at first but slowly progressing to more and more activity. In general, favor activities that build good muscle tone, not those that build great muscle strength. Walking and swimming are better than furniture moving and weight lifting, since tasks requiring a lot of strength put a lot of stress across the joint. And regular exercises done daily are better than occasional sprees of activity that unduly stress joints not ready for so much exertion.

Common sense and a regular, long-term program are the keys to success. Should you take a nap after lunch? Yes, if you're tired. Should you undertake some particular outing? Go on a trip? You know your regular daily activity level. Common sense will answer most such questions. Full normal activity should be approached gradually with a long-term conditioning program that includes rest when needed and gradual increases in activity during non-resting periods.

Physical therapists and occupational therapists can often help with specific advice and helpful hints. The best therapists will help you develop your own program for home exercise and will teach you the exercises and activities that will help your joints. However, don't expect the therapist to do your program for you. Your rest and exercise program cannot consist solely of formal sessions at a rehabilitation facility. You must take the responsibility to build the habits that will, on a daily basis, protect and strengthen your joints. It is important to start exercise and proper use of your joints before you have problems. These are good preventive measures.

Medications are required by almost all patients with rheumatoid arthritis, and often must be continued for years. Great progress has been made recently with disease-modifying antirheumatic drugs (DMARDs), causing a virtual revolution in the treatment of rheumatoid arthritis (see page 277). These crucial drugs should be prescribed early in the course of the disease; the most important rule now is "Don't do too little, too late." At present the DMARD drugs are Plaquenil, Azulfidine, gold shots, oral gold, penicillamine, methotrexate, Imuran, and, in some cases, cyclosporin. More are under development. The great majority of patients with RA should be taking one or a combination of DMARDs at all times.

Aspirin is a valuable drug when used correctly as detailed in Chapter 20. Every patient with RA should become very familiar with the uses of aspirin, which, used correctly, is a good analgesic drug with an acceptable level of side effects. Aspirin variants, such as Disalcid and Trilisate, may better protect the stomach lining. Drugs roughly similar to aspirin are called *nonsteroidal anti-inflammatory drugs* and are also frequently used. Examples of such drugs are Motrin, Voltaren, Naprosyn, Indocin, and Feldene. For more information on these drugs, see Chapter 20.

Antimalarial drugs such as chloroquine or Plaquenil (p. 283) are often used as the first DMARDs. Gold injections (p. 278) are often very helpful and sometimes result in complete disappearance of the arthritis if used early enough. Penicillamine can also result in dramatic improvement. Auranofin (Ridaura) and sulphasalazine (Azulfidine) have been added to this drug category. Both are major advances.

Corticosteroids, most frequently prednisone, are strong hormones with formidable long-term side effects. Their use is controversial in rheumatoid arthritis; some physicians feel that they should almost never be used, while others use them only in very small doses, except in unusual circumstances.

Immunosuppressant drugs such as Imuran (p. 287) or methotrexate (p. 286), are powerful. Methotrexate is now recognized to be the most effective of these strong drugs and is quite well tolerated. Imuran has also proved to be well tolerated by most people, but it is not always as effective. With serious complications, high-dose steroids may be needed but carry substantial risk.

Surgery sometimes can restore the function of a damaged joint. Hip replacement, knee replacement, shoulder replacement, synovectomy of the knee, metatarsal head resection, and synovectomy of the knuckles are among the most frequent operations; these are discussed in Chapter 21.

▼ ▼ ▼ ▼ ▼ ▼ ▼

3. Osteoarthritis: Worn Cartilage

OSTEOARTHRITIS, also known as osteoarthrosis, OA, or degenerative joint disease, DJD, is the kind of arthritis that everybody gets. It is a practically universal problem, increasing with age, and one that, because of its relationship to the aging process, is not as responsive to medical treatment as we might like. However, there are many things you can do for yourself to alleviate this disease. Fortunately, osteoarthritis usually is a relatively mild condition. Osteoarthritis is usually a much less severe form of arthritis than rheumatoid arthritis. In other words, the changes in the skeleton that occur with age are inevitable, but they cause symptoms in a minority of people and severe symptoms in very few.

Osteoarthritis used to be thought of as the inevitable result of "wear and tear." In fact, most activities with a lot of "wear" don't seem to cause much "tear," and authorities now recognize the need for exercise to strengthen the joints, both before and after signs of arthritis have developed. Exercise will very seldom harm someone with OA. Being inactive can cause a great deal of harm.

The tissue involved in osteoarthritis is the cartilage. This is the gristle material that faces the ends of the bones and forms the surface of the joint on both sides. Gristle is tough, somewhat elastic, and very durable. The cartilage or gristle does not have a blood supply, so it gets its oxygen and nutrition from the surrounding joint fluid. In this it is aided by being elastic and by being able to absorb fluid. When we use a joint, the pressure squeezes fluid and waste products out of the cartilage, and when the pressure is relieved, the fluid seeps back, together with oxygen and nutrients. Hence, the health of the cartilage depends on use of the joint. Over many years, the cartilage may become frayed and may even wear away entirely. When this happens, the bone surface on one side of the joint grates against the bone on the other side of the joint, providing a much less elastic joint surface. With time, the opposing bony surfaces may become polished, a process called *eburnation*. As this happens, the joint may again move more smoothly and cause less discomfort. This is one of the reasons it is important to continue to use painful joints.

The difference between the terms *osteoarthritis* and *osteoarthrosis* has to do with the question of inflammation. The suffix *-itis* denotes inflammation, and with osteoarthritis very little inflammation is to be found. Hence, some experts prefer osteoarthrosis, which does not imply inflammation. Otherwise, both words mean the same.

There are three common types of osteoarthritis. The first and mildest causes knobby enlargement of the finger joints. The end joints of the fingers become bony and the hands begin to assume the appearance we associate with old age. The other joints of the fingers may also be involved. This kind of arthritis (or arthrosis) usually causes little difficulty beyond the cosmetic. There may be some stiffness.

The second form of osteoarthritis involves the spine and is sometimes called *degenerative joint disease.* Bony growths (spurs) appear on the spine in the neck region or in the lower back. Usually the bony growths are associated with some narrowing of the space between the vertebrae. This time the disc rather than cartilage is the material that becomes frayed. Changes in the spine begin early in life in almost all of us, but cause symptoms relatively seldom.

The third form of osteoarthritis involves the weight-bearing joints, almost always the hips and knees. These problems can be quite severe. It is possible to have all three kinds of osteoarthritis or any two of them, but often a person will have only one.

Individuals who have had fractures near a joint or have a congenital malformation at a joint seem to develop osteoarthritis in those joints at an earlier age. But, as noted, the usual description of this arthritis as "wear and tear" is not accurate. While excessive wear and tear on the joint can theoretically result in damage, activity helps the joint remain supple and lubricated, and this tends to cancel out the theoretically bad effects.

Careful studies of people who regularly put a lot of stress on joints (such as individuals who operate pneumatic drills or run long distances on hard paved surfaces) have been unable to show a relationship between these activities and the development of arthritis. Hence, intensive activity does not predispose you to arthritis any more than intensive activity predisposes you to heart disease. In fact, the very opposite may be true.

FEATURES

The bony knobs that form around the end joints of the fingers are called *Heberden's nodes* after the British doctor who first described them. In the middle joints of the fingers, similar knobs can be found. Usually, the bony enlargement occurs slowly over a period of years and is not even noticed. In most cases, all of the fingers are involved more or less equally.

Osteoarthritis of the spine does not cause symptoms unless there is pressure on one of the nerves or irritation of some of the other structures of the back. If a doctor tells you that you have arthritis in your spine, do not assume that any pain you feel is necessarily related to that arthritis. Most people with X-rays showing arthritis of the spine do not have any problem at all from the bone spurs seen on the X-ray; the pain is from some nearby structure such as a ligament or muscle.

There is an interesting variation of osteoarthritis in which the bony swelling occurs over only three or four weeks in a single finger joint. The sudden swelling causes redness and soreness until the process is complete; then it stops hurting altogether. This syndrome is seen in women in their forties, earlier than the more usual form of osteoarthritis. These patients frequently have other family members with the same problem. This "familial" form of osteoarthrosis doesn't really seem very much worse over the long run, but one joint after another may suddenly develop a bony knob for a short period of time.

Osteoarthritis of the weight-bearing joints, particularly the hip and knee, develops slowly and often involves both sides of the body. Pain in the joint may remain fairly constant or may wax and wane over a period of years. In severe cases walking may be difficult or even impossible. Fluid may accumulate in the affected joint, giving it a swollen appearance, or a knee may wobble a bit when weight is placed on it. In the knee, the osteoarthritis usually affects the inner or the outer half of the joint more than the other; this may result in the leg becoming bowed or splayed and may cause difficulty walking.

X-rays can be helpful in evaluating osteoarthritis. The two major findings on the X-ray are narrowing of the joint space and the presence of bony spurs, or *osteophytes*. X-rays pass right through cartilage. Hence, in a normal joint the X-ray looks as though the two bones are separated by a space. In reality, the apparent space is filled with cartilage. As the cartilage is frayed, the apparent joint space on the X-ray narrows until the two bones may touch each other. Spurs are little bone growths that appear alongside the places where the cartilage has degenerated. It is as though the body is trying to react to a cartilage problem by providing more surface area for the joint, so as to distribute the weight more evenly. The bony growth provides a larger joint surface, although the new bone is not covered by cartilage. In addition, X-rays can sometimes show the holes through which the nerves pass and can indicate whether these holes are narrowed or not.

Blood tests are not very helpful in diagnosing osteoarthritis. There is nothing wrong with the rest of the body, so all the tests are normal.

PROGNOSIS (WHAT WILL HAPPEN IN THE FUTURE)

Prognosis is good to excellent for all forms of osteoarthritis. When you think of an aging process, you tend to think of a progressive condition that will continue to get worse and worse. That is not necessarily the case. Osteoarthritis may get worse for a while and then become stable for a long time. A joint that has lost its cartilage may not function well at first, but with use the bone may be molded and polished so that a smooth and more functional joint is developed. Even in the worst cases, osteoarthritis progresses slowly. You have lots of time to think about what kinds of treatment are likely to help. If a surgical decision is needed, you can consider for some time whether you want an operation or not. Crippling from osteoarthritis is relatively rare, and most persons with osteoarthritis can remain essentially free of symptoms.

TREATMENT

The revolution in thinking regarding treatment emphasizes the role of exercise. The consequence of osteoarthritis can be loss of physical functional ability. Because of pain, you tend to be less active, and this accelerates the loss of function. People used to be told to "take it easy." Now, it is recognized that even the first symptoms of osteoarthritis are a signal for a regular, dedicated exercise program to increase heart, muscle, ligament, tendon, and bone strength.

Joints should be exercised through their full range of motion several times a day. If weight-bearing joints are involved, body weight should be kept under control; obesity accelerates the rate of damage. The most helpful exercises seem to be swimming, walking, and bicycling, which are easy, can be gradually increased, and are smooth rather than jerky. Exercise should be regular. Thus, if you start getting some osteoarthritis, it is not a signal to begin to tune down your life, but rather to develop a sensible regular exercise program to strengthen the bones and ligaments surrounding the affected joints and to preserve mobility in joints that are developing spurs. (For details on flexibility exercises, see Chapter 11.)

Drug therapy is used to control discomfort. Aspirin in moderate doses is frequently helpful. Recently, acetaminophen (Tylenol), which is the safest analgesic drug, has been found to be just as good for many people as the more toxic (and usually more expensive) alternatives.

Ibuprofen and other anti-inflammatory drugs may be helpful for some people. We try to avoid codeine or other strong pain relievers because pain is a signal to the body that helps protect a diseased joint; it is important that this signal be received. (For details on pain management, see Chapter 15.)

Frequently some kinds of devices can assist. A cane may be helpful; less commonly, crutches are needed. Occasionally, special shoes or lifts on one side of the foot may be helpful.

Most physicians now believe that symptomatic osteoarthritis may be substantially prevented by good health habits. If you are active, maintain a lean body weight, exercise your muscles and joints regularly to nourish cartilage, and let your common sense tell you when you have done too much and something hurts, your joints should last a lifetime. Like exercise of the heart muscle, exercise of the muscles and joints provides reserve for the occasional strenuous activities we all encounter. Exercise builds strong tissues that last a long time.

Injection of osteoarthritic joints with corticosteroids is occasionally helpful, and sometimes removal of some fluid from a joint may help. Usually, however, injections do not help much since there is not much inflammation to be suppressed. Injections should not be frequently repeated, because the injection itself may damage the cartilage and the bone.

Surgery can be dramatically effective for people with severe osteoarthritis of the weight-bearing joints. Total hip replacement is the most important operation yet devised for any form of arthritis. Practically all individuals are free of pain after the surgery and many walk normally and carry out normal activities. Total knee replacement is a more recent operation, one that gives far better results than the knee surgery available just a few years ago. Surgery is never urgent, and you and your doctor will want to decide when the discomfort or the limitation of your walking has become bad enough to warrant the discomfort, costs, and small risk associated with the operation. (For more information on surgery, see Chapter 21.)

4. Osteoporosis: Brittle Bones

OSTEOPOROSIS is a bone disease in which the bones lose calcium, become more brittle, and break more easily. While anyone can have osteoporosis, it is most common in elderly people, particularly women. Because of osteoporosis, one in five women breaks a hip before the age of seventy-five. Inactivity makes osteoporosis worse.

Although the best protection from osteoporosis is prevention, thankfully, we now have some effective treatments for osteoporosis and ideas about ways to prevent it. As with all kinds of arthritis, consistent good health practices are crucial. This starts with a lifestyle that doesn't include smoking, or drinking too much alcohol. The following pages outline the healthy habits that are useful in preventing and dealing with osteoporosis.

DIETARY CALCIUM

Our bones cannot maintain their strength unless our bodies regularly receive an adequate supply of calcium. Recently, the National Institute of Health (NIH) Consensus Development Conference on optimal calcium intake concluded that millions of Americans are not getting nearly enough calcium in their diets and that the official recommended daily allowance (RDA) for calcium may not be adequate for some age groups. The chart on page 20 shows the recommended amounts of calcium for different ages.

To bring your calcium intake up to 800 or 1,000 mg, eat two or three servings of milk products a day (nonfat milk is best) and regularly include other calcium-rich foods in your meals. Also, try to moderate the amount of salt and meat you eat. (Chapter 14 discusses how to do this.) Excessive amounts of sodium or meat can increase your need for calcium.

RECOMMENDED CALCIUM INTAKE

GROUP	OPTIMAL DAILY INTAKE (IN MILLIGRAMS OF CALCIUM)	RDA
Infants		
Birth to 6 months	400 (250 if nursing)	400
6 months to 1 year	600	600
Children 1 to 10 years old	800	800
Teenagers	1,200 to 1,500	1,200
Men		
25 to 50	800	800
51 to 65	1,000	800
Over 65	1,500	800
Women		
25 to 50	1,000	800
Over 50	1,500 (1,000 if taking estrogen)	800
Pregnant and nursing	Additional 400	1,200

The chart "Food Sources of Calcium" gives you a good idea of the types of food that are relatively rich in calcium. Notice that you can get significant quantities of calcium without drinking milk. Yogurts, cheeses, and hot cereals made with milk all supply calcium. Canned salmon, mackerel, and sardines are excellent sources of calcium *if* you eat the soft bones.

FOOD SOURCES OF CALCIUM

FOOD	AMOUNT	CALCIUM (APPROX.)
Low-fat and nonfat milk products		
Nonfat milk	1 cup (235 ml)	300 mg
Low-fat milk (1% fat)	1 cup (235 ml)	300 mg
Low-fat milk (2% fat)	1 cup (235 ml)	295 mg

continued

FOOD SOURCES OF CALCIUM *(continued)*

FOOD	AMOUNT	CALCIUM (APPROX.)
Nonfat dry milk powder	3 tbsp (45 ml)	280 mg
Nonfat yogurt (plain)	1 cup (235 ml)	450 mg
Low-fat yogurt (plain)	1 cup (235 ml)	415 mg
Low-fat cottage cheese (2% fat)	1 cup (235 ml)	155 mg
Part-skim ricotta cheese	1/2 cup (120 ml)	335 mg
Part-skim mozzarella	2 oz (56 g)	365 mg
Full-fat milk products		
Whole milk (3.5% fat)	1 cup (235 ml)	290 mg
Whole-milk yogurt (plain)	1 cup (235 ml)	275 mg
Swiss cheese	1 oz (28 g)	270 mg
Processed Swiss cheese	1 oz (28 g)	220 mg
Cheddar cheese	1 oz (28 g)	205 mg
Processed American cheese	1 oz (28 g)	125 mg
Ice milk (hard, not soft-serve)	1 cup (235 ml)	175 mg
Ice cream (regular, 10% fat)	1 cup (235 ml)	175 mg
Ice cream (rich, 16% fat)	1 cup (235 ml)	150 mg
Other calcium-rich foods		
Almonds	1 oz (28 g)	75 mg
Broccoli (boiled)	1 cup (235 ml)	180 mg
Corn tortilla	1	40 mg
Great northern beans (boiled)	1 cup (235 ml)	120 mg
Kale (boiled)	1 cup (235 ml)	95 mg
Navy beans (boiled)	1 cup (235 ml)	130 mg
Pinto beans (boiled)	1 cup (235 ml)	80 mg
Tofu (soybean curd)	1/2 cup (120 ml)	130 mg
Canned jack mackerel (including bones)	1/2 cup (120 ml)	230 mg
Canned salmon (including bones)	3 oz (84 g)	190 mg
Canned sardines (including bones)	1 oz (28 g)	85 mg

For most people, low-fat and nonfat dairy products are better choices than full-fat products. See Chapter 14.

Supplemental Calcium

It is better to get calcium from your foods than to rely on calcium supplements. But if you cannot eat two or more servings of dairy products every day, or if you want to take in more than 1,000 mg of calcium, supplements can provide practical help.

Chapter 14 explains how to choose a calcium supplement and notes some important precautions to observe. In general, choose a supplement that contains between 500 and 1,000 mg (50% to 100% of the RDA) of "elemental calcium." "Elemental calcium" means the actual amount of calcium in the pill. Take one or two full doses a day, depending on your needs, not more.

As the charts illustrate, the elemental calcium in a supplement can come from any of several different calcium compounds. Less expensive store-brand supplements are usually fine; use the product that suits you best. Sometimes inexpensive calcium tablets won't dissolve in your stomach, however, so try this test. Put a tablet in half a glass of water for thirty minutes. It should become shaggy and partly dissolve. If not, fill the glass the rest of the way with vinegar, stir gently, and wait another half hour. If the tablet is still not dissolved, it is not a good product for you.

SUPPLEMENTAL CALCIUM	
SOURCES OF SUPPLEMENTAL CALCIUM	ELEMENTAL CALCIUM CONTENT
Calcium carbonate (in oyster-shell calcium, BioCal, Caltrate 600, OsCal, Tums)	40%
Calcium citrate (in CitraCal)	21%
Calcium lactate (available in store-brand products)	13%

Myths About Calcium

1. "Calcium causes bone spurs." Maintaining a calcium intake of 800 to 1,500 mg a day (or even much higher) will not cause bone spurs.
2. "Calcium causes kidney stones." While it is prudent to avoid calcium intakes that exceed 2,000 to 2,500 mg a day, consuming a total of 800 to 1,500 mg a day is unlikely to lead to kidney stones. If you have had kidney stones in the past, you should check with your doctor before starting a calcium supplement. Otherwise, just be sure to drink plenty of fluids whenever you take a calcium tablet.

3. "Calcium causes constipation." Large doses of calcium can cause constipation in some people. But the problem generally can be avoided by drinking plenty of fluids and eating foods high in fiber. See Chapter 14 for more information.

HORMONES

Calcium by itself will not stop bone loss. The body needs a stimulus to absorb the calcium and to get it into the bone. The two best stimuli are estrogen therapy for postmenopausal women and adequate weight-bearing exercise for everybody. The use of hormones such as estrogen after menopause has long been a topic of controversy. This is a subject every woman should discuss with her physician. The following discussion is to help you understand some of the issues.

Estrogen

There are two female hormones, estrogen and progestin. These hormones are normally created during the menstrual cycle. After menopause, their levels fall greatly. Taking supplemental estrogen after menopause seems to protect against osteoporosis. However, it is believed by some to increase the likelihood of endometrial cancer (cancer of the lining of the uterus). When progesterone is taken with the estrogen, this risk is greatly reduced. The decision to take no hormone, one hormone (either estrogen or progestin), or a combination of the two is a personal one and should be discussed with a physician. The correct treatment is still in debate, but more and more physicians are recommending estrogens for postmenopausal women.

Calcitonin

The only currently approved alternative to estrogen-replacement therapy for treatment of osteoporosis is salmon calcitonin. The major drawback to the treatment is its expense and the necessity for patients to learn self-administered injections. The medication may cause transient flushing and nausea in about 20% of patients. Other forms of calcitonin administration such as nasal spray and suppositories are under study.

Other Treatments Under Study

Etidronate (Didronel) belongs to a class of drugs called bisphosphonates, and has been shown to produce a small increase in spine bone density and to decrease the short-term incidence of spine fractures. It is given daily for two weeks every three months. Because it is poorly absorbed, it must be taken on an empty stomach and only with water. Long-term efficacy is still under investigation. Other studies evaluating the efficacy and safety of medications such as low-dose fluoride, growth factors, and parathyroid hormones are under way for treatment of osteoporosis.

EXERCISE

Weight-bearing exercise is most important in maintaining strong bones. The body reacts to such exercise by increasing the calcium content and thus the strength of the bones. Walking is the best example. If at all possible, walk half a mile to a mile (1 to 1½ km) a day. Even if this is unrealistic for you, remember that even a little weight-bearing exercise is important. Do as much as you can. For suggestions on developing a walking program, see Chapters 10 and 13. Recent research has shown that women need to walk four miles (6 km) a week to get maximal exercise benefit for osteoporosis prevention. This includes all the walking we do in our daily lives. (Note: Swimming is *not* a weight-bearing exercise.)

PREVENTING FALLS

Unfortunately, it is not always possible to prevent osteoporosis or undo damage already done. Thus, avoiding falls is very important to prevent broken bones. The following are a few hints:

▼ Avoid area rugs—they are slippery and have a bad habit of tripping the unwary.

▼ Be sure all stairs have a secure railing that is easy to grasp.

▼ If advised to do so by a health professional, use a cane, stick, or walker. These can be real bone savers.

▼ Even if you don't usually use a cane, consider using one for getting up at night. This is a time when most of us may easily lose our balance and a cane can help prevent bad spills.

▼ Watch for uneven walks, curbs, floors, and so on.

▼ Move the phone to a convenient place so you won't trip over the cord.

▼ Wear shoes that give good support.

▼ Use step stools that are stable and in good repair.

▼ Use nonskid mats in the bathtub and shower, and on the bathroom floor. Permanently install grab bars to wall or edge of tub.

▼ If you are unsteady on your feet, sit on a stool with nonskid feet when showering or bathing.

▼ Have light switches at the top and bottom of all stairs.

▼ Be careful not to hold your breath when you are on the toilet. This can cause you to pass out and fall.

SUMMARY: PREVENTING AND TREATING OSTEOPOROSIS

There are five things you can do to help prevent and treat osteoporosis:

1. Make positive lifestyle changes: Stop smoking, reduce alcohol consumption.
2. Do some weight-bearing exercises daily.
3. Using diet or a combination of diet and supplements, take adequate calcium.
4. If advised by your physician, take estrogen, progestin, or a combination of these hormones.
5. Make your home and other surroundings fall-safe.

▼ ▼ ▼ ▼ ▼ ▼ ▼

5. *Fibromyalgia: Chronic Pain and Fatigue*

*F*IBROMYALGIA is a common and increasingly recognized condition. In 1990 it was defined in terms of two distinguishing characteristics:

▼ Pain and aching in many parts of the body lasting for at least 3 months
▼ Local tenderness in eleven of eighteen specified places on the body

FEATURES

The fibromyalgia syndrome (FMS) is a very common condition, affecting perhaps five million people in the United States alone and accounting for one out of every six visits to rheumatologists. Patients are more likely to be women, but children, the elderly, and men can also be affected. Their average age is about fifty-five. People with this syndrome also may experience sleep disturbances, severe fatigue, morning stiffness, irritable bowel syndrome, anxiety, and other symptoms, such as trouble remembering things.

The *tender points* are particular body locations that are normally somewhat tender; many readers will be able to identify these points on their own bodies. Firm pressure applied to these areas will hurt anyone, but the person with fibromyalgia experiences great pain when these areas are pressed lightly. For example, about halfway between the neck and the shoulder, one can feel the upper border of the trapezius muscle; at the midpoint of this muscle there is a tender site. The "tennis elbow" site is just about an inch (2.5 cm) down the forearm from the outer bump on the side of the elbow when the palm is turned up; this tender spot may feel like a cord. There is also tenderness at the second costochondral junction, next to the breastbone on either side and about an inch or two (2 to 5 cm) below the collarbone. A fourth site is in the fat pad on the inside portion of the knee. Others are between the shoulder blades and at the base of the skull. A person with fibromyalgia usually has tenderness at most of these places and may have widespread tenderness as well.

Half or more of those with fibromyalgia have chronic fatigue. Fatigue may be severe and interfere with activities. Some of the factors which contribute to fatigue are pain, sleep problems, and stress factors. A frequent but not quite universal characteristic of fibromyalgia is sleep disturbance. There is an interruption of slow-wave brain activity, the kind of sleep most restful to the muscles, in many patients. Patients frequently report that upon awakening in the morning they feel as though they never got to sleep at all.

Although the cause of fibromyalgia is unknown, researchers have several theories about causes or triggers of the disease. There is elevation of a pain peptide (substance P) in the cerebrospinal fluid; it may be that there is a new "thermostat" setting for the pain threshold in fibromyalgia patients. Serotonin in the platelets is lower than normal. Fibromyalgia may be associated with changes in muscle metabolism such as decreased blood flow, causing fatigue and decreased strength. Others believe that the syndrome may be triggered by an infectious agent, such as a virus, in susceptible people. Stress is also a frequently reported cause.

We recommend an excellent book, *The Fibromyalgia Handbook,* by Jenny Fransen and I. Jon Russell (Smith House Press, St. Paul, MN). A superb video is available through Fibromyalgia Information Resources, P.O. Box 690402, San Antonio, TX 78269.

PROGNOSIS (WHAT WILL HAPPEN IN THE FUTURE)

Medically, fibromyalgia carries a fairly good prognosis for most people. There will usually be no crippling, but the discomfort may last for many years or even for life. The pain can vary over a period of months or years but often never fully goes away. In the U.S. most fibromyalgia patients are able to work. About 30% have had to reduce the duration or physical exertion associated with their jobs. About 15% are disabled and receiving Social Security disability payments.

Fibromyalgia symptoms may also be seen in many other disease conditions, such as rheumatoid arthritis, lupus, or Sjogren's syndrome, which themselves may disturb sleep. The "secondary" fibromyalgia must not be confused with a flare-up of the other condition, since the treatment is different.

TREATMENT

Exercise, slowly increased toward full aerobic cardiovascular conditioning and physical tiredness, is the single most important component of treatment. Start slowly; even a minute or two an hour is helpful if you have been completely inactive. For more help with exercise, see Chapter 10. When a patient is able to walk extensively and to swim, hike, or bicycle regularly, we sometimes have seen gradual resolution of the problem in only a few months. In general, impact exercises such as jogging, tennis, or basketball should be avoided. Stretching exercises are important. Pain often gets somewhat worse with a new exercise program before it gets better. Studies have shown that aerobic exercise improves muscle fitness and reduces muscle pain and tenderness. It may also improve sleep.

Progressive muscle relaxation or some other structured relaxation program may also be helpful (see Chapter 15). Heat and massage may give short-term relief. Pain management programs may be beneficial; the most success has come from psychological interventions which include cognitive behavioral therapy. Check with your local chapter of The Arthritis Foundation or The Arthritis Society for information about fibromyalgia support groups.

Medications which have been proven most effective are generally given an hour before bed time and have included amitriptyline (Elavil), cyclobenzaprine (Flexeril), alprazolam (Xanax), and Soma. While these drugs have anti-depressive properties, they are not given for depression, but to improve sleep quality and to relax muscles. These medications increase deep (stage 4) sleep. Ordinary "sleeping pills" are generally not helpful. Non-steroidal drugs such as ibuprofen or naproxen are often used, with variable success. An increasingly common regimen is Prozac in the morning and Elavil in the evening. Side effects of medications are common but can often be avoided by use of lower doses and by changing the timing of the dose. Some authorities recommend vitamin B_1 and B_6 supplements, and benefit has been reported with a combination of magnesium and malic acid.

6. Other Nagging Pains

Most of the problems we tend to call arthritis don't involve the joints and really aren't even diseases. This is good news. Painful local conditions involving only one or two parts of the body are almost always just an irritation or injury of that part. After that part is rested or fixed, everything is all right again. There is no crippling, no threat to life, no need for dangerous medications. Remember the basic principle: For a local problem use a local treatment. Very seldom will you want to take a medication by mouth for pain in, say, an elbow.

There are a lot of names for these conditions—bursitis, lower-back strain, sciatica, metatarsalgia, Achilles tendinitis, heel-spur syndrome, sprained ankle, cervical neck strain, frozen shoulder, tennis elbow, housemaid's knee, carpal tunnel syndrome, and others. Many people call all of these "bursitis," while doctors have other and fancier names for them. But they are all local conditions and are approached the same way. At first you don't even need a doctor for them, but if they don't respond after six weeks of self-treatment or seem alarmingly severe, be sure to see the doctor.

BURSITIS: INFLAMED BURSAE

A bursa is a small sac of tissue similar to the synovial tissue that lines the joints. The bursa sac contains a lubricating fluid, and the bursa is designed to ease the movement of muscle across muscle or muscle across bone. A bursa does not connect to the joint space of the nearby joint but is a separate sac. In the grand scheme of things the bursa is just an annoying little body area, but bursae can be very painful when they become inflamed. Usually, only one or two will be inflamed at a time, but bursitis of over twenty bursae can occur, and the problems can come and go over the years.

"Housemaid's knee" is an outdated term for *prepatellar bursitis,* in which the bursa in front and just below the kneecap is inflamed. *Olecranon bursitis* occurs over the point of the elbow, and sometimes a fluid-filled sac is visible at that point. *Subdeltoid bursitis* occurs at the shoulder, or more precisely, on the outer part of the upper arm just below the shoulder.

Features

Bursitis is inflammation of a bursa and results in localized pain. Sometimes the pain is on both sides of the body, as with both knees. There is pain when the inflamed area is pressed, and heat and redness are common. If the bursa is located close enough to the skin, swelling can be seen. Many bursae, however, are buried deep between muscles.

Bursitis comes on relatively suddenly, from within hours to days. It frequently follows injury to the area, repeated pressure on the area, or overuse. In the shoulders, particularly, it may be associated with inflammation of the tendon and can be part of a "frozen shoulder" problem.

Prognosis

Almost all episodes of bursitis will subside within several days to several weeks, but may recur. If the process causing the bursitis is continued, the bursitis may persist, otherwise it follows a normal healing course over a period of seven to ten days. Some people seem more prone to bursitis than others and have recurrent problems throughout their lives. If the affected part is held rigid, some permanent stiffness may result; otherwise no crippling whatsoever should result from bursitis.

Treatment

If the problem is tolerable, treat it with "tincture of time." Wait for the body to control and heal the process. Avoid the precipitating cause. Use drugs very sparingly; the process is local, so systemic drugs like aspirin are not very helpful. Resting the part will speed the healing, and you may want to use a sling or other device to increase the rest. Gentle warmth provided by a heating pad or warm bath frequently makes the bursitis feel better. Additional techniques described in Chapter 11 may also be helpful.

Patience and avoidance of reinjury are the major tactics, but you should remain active. The affected area should be worked through its full range of motion two to four times a day, even if it is a bit tender, to prevent stiffness from developing. Continue to exercise other parts of the body regularly.

If the discomfort persists for a number of weeks despite the measures outlined above, see the doctor. Often, the doctor will recommend that you continue the same general measures discussed here. Alternatively, an anti-inflammatory drug may be prescribed; these help few people and are generally just a way of buying a little more patience from the patient. Finally, the doctor may inject the bursa with corticosteroids (see Chapter 20). These injections are usually successful and not overly painful. They are relatively free of side effects and most physicians feel that they are appropriate treatment for a local condition that is severe and persistent.

LOWER-BACK SYNDROMES

Pain in the lower back has been called the "curse of the erect posture." From an engineering standpoint, when humans developed a standing posture, the spine developed a double bend, concave in the lower back and convex in the upper back. The back is a complex mechanism with hundreds of ligaments and scores of joints; it should not be surprising that injury to this complicated organ occurs in over one half of all people. Pain can be extremely severe and has been compared with the pain of childbirth, kidney stones, or a heart attack. Lower-back pain results in as much long-term disability and as many days lost from work as does almost any other illness or injury. Yet as we will see, it is always difficult to be sure what is going on in any individual case.

The spine consists of a stack of bones, the *vertebrae*. Each vertebra is connected to the next one by ligaments that cross the vertebral disks. The disks separate the bones much like mushrooms on a shish kebab. Long ligaments run up and down the length of the spine. Muscles attach each vertebra to the ones directly adjacent; other muscles bridge two vertebrae, and three, and four, and so forth. In addition to the disks separating the vertebrae, there are small joints that provide two additional points of contact and movement. These small joints are bridged by ligaments and have synovial tissue within them just like larger joints.

Problems with the disk itself will be discussed in the following section; most lower-back syndromes, however, are due to problems with one of the back parts mentioned above—the ligaments, the muscles, the joint synovium, or the joint ligaments. Additionally, obese people may have little ruptures of fat through the back tissues and pain from that event.

All minor injuries of the back look and act about the same. A major disk problem, a *herniated nucleus pulposis*, is different and may involve nerve injury. From the outside, neither the doctor nor the patient can tell exactly which tissue was initially injured. Wherever the problem started, a larger portion of the back becomes involved as the body works to immobilize the part to allow its healing. In such cases, muscle spasm and widespread pain are the rule.

Features

Lower-back syndromes usually result from an injury. The injury is usually obvious, but in at least one third of patients no incident can be remembered. Muscle spasm provides protection for the injured part by helping to immobilize the back, but this spasm is itself painful. Except for the spasm, which is unique to the back, think of a lower-back problem as analogous to the more familiar sprain of an ankle. The pain and local swelling are maximum within 24 hours, remain acute and severe for 24 to 72 hours, are somewhat nagging for another week, and require perhaps six weeks to heal back to full strength. Reinjury is very common and starts the timetable all over again. Frequent reinjury can lead to chronic sprains that are more difficult to treat and take a longer time to heal.

The pain is usually most pronounced in the concave portion of the lower back and may frequently radiate to the buttocks. There is pain in the areas of muscle spasm, and on subsequent days, the pain may rise higher in the back as the tired muscles that have been in spasm begin to complain loudly. The pain should not go down into the calf; if it does run down a leg, it is a reason to see the doctor.

The most frequent injury is a sudden hyperextension, in which the lower body continues forward and the upper body is suddenly arched backward. However, all kinds of injuries can result in these syndromes. Injuries occur most frequently in the overweight or inactive individual, or in the individual who exercises only episodically. Good muscle tone and regular exercise protect the back and decrease the risk of these conditions.

Prognosis

About half of patients with lower-back syndromes have only one to three episodes over a lifetime; the remainder have more episodes than this. Prognosis for the individual episode is excellent, and the chances of a serious problem involving pressure on nerves or requiring spinal surgery are less than 1%. If the pain runs down into the legs, particularly the outside of the legs and particularly below the knee, the prognosis is more guarded, and greater care in management and in the consideration of surgery is necessary.

If the pain is somewhat less dramatic but lasts for a period of many weeks or months, is worst in the morning, is rather slow in developing, gets better with exercise during the day, and occurs in a person below age 40, ankylosing spondylitis, discussed earlier, should be suspected. Common lower-back syndromes may loosen up a little bit with activity, but by and large they get worse if you overdo before the healing is complete.

Treatment

The primary goal in treating an acute lower-back problem is to prevent it from becoming chronic. The injury must heal and this takes time. For the acute painful problem, two possible treatment strategies are acceptable. A third one is not. First, there is the "least pain" way. This involves bed rest, a bed board to provide firm support, sometimes a small pillow beneath the lower back if this increases comfort, heat beginning the second day, and pain relievers and muscle relaxants as required to provide comfort.

The second is the "natural" way, in which the patient is up and around as the pain allows, avoids pain relievers, and does not use muscle relaxants. The body will heal this problem if left alone.

The third (and unacceptable) way is the "reinjury" way, in which the patient *both* is up and around *and* uses pain relievers and muscle relaxants. If you blunt the pain response of the body and interfere with the immobilization provided naturally by muscle spasm, then reinjury is likely and will delay healing.

You can prevent reinjury by greatly limiting activity—this is the "least pain" way. Or you can prevent reinjury by allowing the pain reflex and the muscle spasm to protect the injured point—this is the "natural" way. But if you combine these strategies, you are asking for a long-term problem.

After the acute injury is over, it is time to begin thinking about preventing the next one. Control of weight involves not only reducing to a good body weight but also constant maintenance of that weight. Development of gentle, regular, graded activity to strengthen the spine and improve muscle tone is important. Back protection techniques can help prevent injury when lifting or using the back for different tasks. And specific back exercises can help to strengthen the muscles on the outside of the back and also those that are inside and unseen. By gradually increasing activity, most patients with lower-back syndromes can return to any activity desired. Even horseback riding and heavy labor are entirely possible if the progression to full activity is patient and gradual.

CARPAL TUNNEL SYNDROME

The carpal tunnel syndrome is a malady so common that most of us get it, at least briefly, at some point. Most of the time it is not serious or even very troublesome. But sometimes it is. The word *carpal* means "wrist." The wrist is a surprisingly complex place, with a bunch of little bones held together by ligaments. On the palm side of the wrist are the blood vessels to the hand, as well as the median nerve. To keep them from bulging out, there is a stout band of fibrous tissue going across the front of the wrist, leaving a tunnel beneath. This is the carpal tunnel. The blood vessels and median nerve go through it.

The problem is that injury to the median nerve can occur in the carpal tunnel. This is the "carpal tunnel syndrome." Basically this occurs in one of two ways. The most common cause is trauma, in which repetitive movements involving full motion at the wrist actually irritate the nerve by causing the fibrous band to hit against the nerve surface. The second cause is that with inflammatory forms of arthritis (and some other medical conditions) you can have swelling within the carpal tunnel. The swollen tissue can compress the median nerve and prevent its proper function. This is the more serious form.

Features

The first symptom is numbness in the fingers, resulting from compression of the median nerve. Here, if you are careful, you can make a very accurate diagnosis at home. The key point is to notice which fingers are numb. The median nerve sends nerve fibers to the thumb, the first finger, and the middle finger. Usually it sends fibers to the middle finger side of the ring finger as well, but not always. It almost never sends nerve fibers to the little finger. Thus, to make the diagnosis, you need to very carefully pay attention to which fingers are numb. If the little finger is not numb but there is numbness in the other fingers, then it is the carpal tunnel syndrome. Even better, sometimes you can tell a difference in the sensation by stroking the ring finger on both sides. If the ring finger is only one half numb (the half closest to the middle finger), you can be certain of the diagnosis.

There are two other frequently used tests. If you tap on the inside of your wrist with the middle finger of the other hand you may notice a tingling, like hitting your funny bone. The tingling goes down into your fingers. Again, this will not involve the little finger but will involve the thumb, first, and middle fingers. If you can cause the tingling by tapping over the carpal tunnel, then you have the carpal tunnel syndrome. Another test is to bend both wrists in as far as they will go, then touch the back sides of your hands to each other, so that both hands are at a right angle to the arms with the fingers pointing down. Hold them this way for three to five minutes. This puts pressure on the median nerve and if you have the carpal tunnel syndrome, this may make the symptoms come on. Most of the time people really don't need fancy medical tests to establish whether or not they have carpal tunnel syndrome. You can suspect the problem strongly by the time you go to see the doctor.

Prognosis

What can happen from the carpal tunnel syndrome if it is not treated? Most of the time, not very much, but the pain and numbness can be continual and quite aggravating. If it does persist for too long, there is some chance of permanent nerve damage, and you may develop weakness of the thumb muscles, which also get nerve fibers from the median nerve.

Treatment

What to do? First, if the problem results from a repetitive activity that uses a lot of wrist motion, you need to avoid that activity. Second, you can put wrist splints, available at most large drug stores or hospital supply stores, on each arm at night; this will provide rest for the wrists so that the inflammation within the carpal tunnel can decrease and your symptoms can get better or disappear.

If neither of these simple things work, an injection of a long-acting corticosteroid medication by a physician can reduce the swelling and in most instances greatly improve the symptoms. This is quite a simple procedure and is usually effective. If all else fails, a surgeon can cut the carpal tunnel band and release the excess pressure so that you get relief.

In sum, the carpal tunnel syndrome is a mysterious-sounding condition which is actually quite simple, and usually not too serious.

GETTING OLD

Local injuries, like bursitis, are often dismissed as "just getting old, I guess." It is true that more older people than younger people have these problems, and they do have something to do with the way our bodies age.

But they do not need to happen. These problems are sometimes due to abuse of a body part, as in the traditional prepatellar bursitis from scrubbing floors on your knees. Much more frequently, however, they are due to lack of use. In our society, as you get older you are expected to be less active. And then you get the kinds of health problems that happen to inactive people of all ages. The relationship between local problems and age is mostly accidental; it is really an association of local problems with inactivity.

So you need to be active. If your muscles are trim and in good tone, your heart and lungs are conditioned, your body weight is normal and constant at that level, and you have a regular exercise program, you will have far fewer of these problems, and your body will not grow old as rapidly. These measures will keep calcium in your bones, your bursae free and well lubricated, your tendons firm and strong, and your joint cartilage well nourished.

You can control a lot of the aging of your body. The worst mistake you can make is to consider bursitis or another local problem to be a signal to slow down. It is a signal to speed up, because your body is drifting out of condition. In Chapters 10, 12, and 13 we go through some of the exercises that can help.

▼ ▼ ▼ ▼ ▼ ▼ ▼ ▼ ▼ ▼

PART TWO

Your Self-Management Plan

7. Becoming an Arthritis Self-Manager

SELF-MANAGEMENT seems like a simple enough term, yet it needs some explaining. Both at home and in the business world the managers direct the show. They don't do everything themselves; they work with others, including consultants, to get the job done. What makes them managers is that they are responsible for making the decisions and making sure that these decisions are carried through. As an *arthritis self-manager*, your job is much the same. You gather information from friends, family, the Arthritis Foundation or Arthritis Society, and written materials. You hire a consultant or a team of consultants: your physician, physical therapist, pharmacists, and other health professionals. Once they have given you their best advice, it is up to you to follow through.

Arthritis, like diabetes and other chronic diseases, needs to be managed. Cures are usually not possible. However, your quality of life, and how you are affected by the disease, is very much up to you. Have you noticed that some people with severe physical problems get on very well, while others with lesser problems seem to give up on life? The difference is management style.

Being a good manager means working with others, discussing problems, and, most important, understanding that the management is a day-to-day job. This doesn't mean that all your decisions will be correct. Managing arthritis, like managing a family, is a complex undertaking. There are many twists, turns, and midcourse corrections. By learning self-management skills you can ease the problems of living with arthritis.

The key to success in any undertaking is first learning a set of skills and then practicing them until they have been mastered. Children cannot read without first learning to recognize the letters of the alphabet. They then learn the sounds of combinations of letters. Later, they learn the meanings of simple words and phrases. It is only after years of practice and mastery that one is able to read a novel. Think about it. The same is true with almost everything we do, from baking a cake to driving a car to planting a garden. These tasks are all based on learning skills and mastering them. Success in arthritis self-management is the same. One needs to learn a set of skills and then to practice them daily until success is reached.

This book is full of information about skills that can help relieve some of the problems caused by arthritis. However, we have learned that knowing the skills is not enough. Most of us need a way of incorporating these skills into our daily lives. Unfortunately, whenever we try a new skill, the first attempts are clumsy and slow, and show few results. It is easier to return to our old ways than to continue to try to master new and sometimes difficult skills. One of the best ways to master new skills is through goal setting. In the following pages, we will try to outline some of the principles of goal setting. If you use these principles, the success of an arthritis self-management program is almost assured.

In arthritis, you are your own manager. Like any manager of an organization or household, you must do the following:

1. Decide what you want to accomplish (your long-term **goal**).

2. Determine the necessary **steps** to accomplish this goal.

3. Start making short-term plans (**contracts** with yourself).

4. **Carry out** your contracts.

5. **Check** the results.

6. Make midcourse **corrections** as needed.

GOALS

Deciding what you want to accomplish may be the easiest part of being a manager. Think of all the things you would like to do. One of our self-managers wanted to climb twenty steps to her daughter's home so she could join her family for a holiday meal. Another wanted to lose weight so he could receive a hip replacement. Still another wanted to be more socially active. In each case the goal was one that would take several weeks or even months to accomplish. In fact, one of the problems with goals is they often seem more like dreams. They are so far off that we don't even try to accomplish them. However, a good management program starts (but does not end) with goals. Take a moment now and write your goals here.

GOALS

1. _____
2. _____
3. _____

STEPS

There are many different ways to reach any specific goal. For example, our self-manager who wanted to climb twenty steps could start off with a slow-walking program, knee-strengthening exercises, learning how to use a cane, or starting to climb a few stairs each day. The man who wanted to lose weight could decide not to eat between meals, to give up desserts, to cut down on fried foods, or to start an exercise program. The self-manager who wanted more social contact could find out about community college classes, church groups, or other organizations, or could call or write friends, or maybe find out about organized trips. She could call the Arthritis Foundation or Arthritis Society to find out about support groups, exercise classes, or volunteer opportunities.

As you can see, there are many options for reaching each goal. The job here is to list the options and then choose one or two on which you would like to work. Write the options for each of your goals here. Put a star next to those on which you would like to work: If you cannot think of any options, share your goal with friends, family, or health professionals and ask for suggestions. Remember, self-managers use consultants.

OPTIONS

1. _____
2. _____
3. _____
4. _____
5. _____

CONTRACTS

A short-term plan, which we will call a contract, calls for a specific action that you can realistically expect to accomplish within the next week. This is probably your most important self-management tool. Most of us can do things that would make us healthier but often fail to do them. For example, most people with arthritis can walk: some just across the room, others for half a block. Most can walk several blocks, and some can walk a mile (1¹/₂ km) or more. However, few people have a systematic exercise program, even though they know it would be good for them. A contract helps us to do the things we know we should. Let us go through all the steps for making a realistic contract. This is a very important skill and may well determine the success of your self-management program.

First, decide what you will do this week. For our step climber this might be climbing three steps on four days. The man trying to lose weight may decide not to eat between meals for three days. This action must be something that you want to do, that you feel you realistically can do, and that is a step on the way to your long-term goal.

Then make a specific plan. This is the most difficult and important part of making a contract. Deciding what you want to do is worthless without a plan to do it. The plan should contain all of the following steps.

1. Exactly what is it that you are going to do? For example, how far will you walk, how will you eat less, what pain-management technique will you practice?

2. How much will you do? For example, walk around the block, walk for fifteen minutes, climb three stairs, write letters to two friends.

3. When will you do this? Again, this must be specific: before lunch; in the shower; when I come home from work. Connecting a new activity with an old habit is a good way to be sure it gets done.

4. How often will you do the activity? This is a bit tricky. We would all like to do things every day. However, we are human and this is not always possible. It is usually best to contract to do something three or four times a week. If you do more, so much the better. However, if you are like most of us, you can do your activity three or four times and still succeed at your contract.

In writing your contract there are a couple of guidelines that may help you toward success. First, start where you are or start slowly. If you can walk around the block, start your walking program with walking around the block, not with walking a kilometer or a mile. If you have never done any exercise for arthritis, start with just a few minutes of warm-up, endurance, and cool-down exercises. A total of five to ten minutes is enough. Some people may start by walking one minute an hour. If you want to lose weight, set a goal based on your eating behaviors, such as not eating after dinner.

See Chapter 10 for help in starting an exercise program and Chapter 14 for more information on diet and nutrition.

Also, give yourself some time off. All people have days when they don't feel like doing anything. Therefore, it is best to say that you will do something three to five times a week but not every day. That way, if you don't feel like walking one day, you can still meet your contract.

Once you've made your contract, ask yourself the following question: "On a scale of 0 to 10, with 0 being totally unsure and 10 being totally certain, how certain am I that I can complete all of this contract?"

If your answer is 7 or above, this is probably a realistic contract. Congratulate yourself, you have done the hard work. If your answer is below 7, then you should reassess your contract. Ask yourself what makes you uncertain. What problems do you foresee? Then see if you can either solve the problems or change your contract to make yourself more certain of success.

Once you have made a contract you are happy with, write it down on a contract form or calendar and post this sheet where you will see it every day. Keep track of how you are doing and the problems you encounter. Page 46 is an example of a contract sheet. You may want to make copies of this, since you will be making contracts weekly.

CARRYING OUT YOUR CONTRACT

If the contract is well-written and realistic, fulfilling it is generally pretty easy. Ask family or friends to check with you on how you are doing. Having to report your progress is good motivation. While carrying out your plan, keep track of your daily activities. All good managers have lists of what they want to accomplish, and check things off as they are completed. This will give you guidance on how realistic your planning was, and will also be useful in making future plans. Make daily notes, even of the things you don't understand at the time. Later, these notes may be useful in establishing a pattern which can be used for problem solving.

For example, our stair-climbing friend never did her climbing. Each day, she had a different problem: not enough time, being tired, the weather being too cold, and so on. When she looked back at this, she began to realize that the real problem was that she was afraid that she might fall with no one around to help her. She then decided to use a cane while climbing stairs and to do it when a friend or neighbor was around.

CHECKING THE RESULTS

At the end of each week, see if you are any nearer to accomplishing your goal. Are you able to walk farther? Have you lost weight? Are you less fatigued? Taking stock is important. You may not see progress day by day, but you should see a little progress each week. If your contract involves exercise, you can use some of the self-tests in Chapters 11–13. Also, at the end of each week, check on how well you have fulfilled your contract. If you are having problems, this is a good time to use consultants. Depending on the problem, consultants may be friends, family, or members of your health-care team. Remember, consultants never solve your problems. They only help you accomplish your goal.

CORRECTIONS

In any business, the first plan is not always the workable plan. If something doesn't work, don't give up. Try something else. Modify your short-term plans so that your steps are easier. Give yourself more time to accomplish difficult tasks. Choose new steps to your goal, or check with your consultants for their advice and aid.

If you run into problems, don't stop; get help. For example, one self-manager we know was going to walk with a coworker every day at lunch. The problem was that even though the coworker tried to slow down, she walked too fast. The solution was simple. The woman asked her coworker to always walk slightly behind her. Thus, the self-manager set the pace and was able to continue on her daily walk.

Another self-manager wanted to tell her grown children that hosting big holiday dinners had just become too much for her. However, she didn't know how to do this. By talking to friends, she first decided to offer to cook the turkey and have the children each bring a dish and clean up. Then, she rehearsed saying, "I know how much of a tradition holiday dinners are. However, I just can't do as much anymore. I'll cook the turkey, and will you each bring something?" This story had a happy ending, as the children had all wanted to help for years but had not offered for fear of offending their mother. Chapters 15–18 can help you with problem solving.

For some problems, consultants can be most helpful. If medications are causing problems, ask the advice of your physician. If you just stop taking the drug, you are cheating yourself in two ways. First, you are not getting the benefits of medication. Second, you have not supplied your consultant with the vital information he or she needs to help you manage successfully.

If you really enjoy swimming, but have problems because you cannot comfortably turn your head, check with an occupational therapist. You probably don't need ongoing treatment, but one problem-solving visit with a professional may keep you in the water. (In this case the solution might be a face mask and snorkel.)

The best part of being a good self-manager is the rewards you will get in accomplishing your goals. However, don't wait until your goal is attained; reward yourself frequently. For example, decide that you won't read the paper until after you exercise. Thus, reading the paper becomes your reward. One self-manager (she is one of this book's authors) buys only one or two pieces of fruit at a time and walks the half mile to the supermarket every day or two to get more fruit. Rewards don't have to be fancy or expensive, just something that is pleasant and meaningful in your life.

To review, a successful self-manager does the following:

1. Sets goals
2. Determines what is necessary to carry out the goal
3. Makes short-term plans or contracts
4. Carries out the contract
5. Checks on progress weekly
6. Makes midcourse corrections as necessary

REFERENCES

Lewis, Kathleen. *Successful Living with Chronic Illness: Celebrating the Joys of Life.* Dubuque, Iowa: Kendall/Hunt Publishing, 1994.

Lorig, K., Holman, H., Sobel, D., Laurent, D., González, V., & Minor, M. *Living a Healthy Life with Chronic Conditions.* Palo Alto, Calif.: Bull Publishing Co., 1994.

CONTRACT FORM

When you write a contract, be sure it includes

1. **What** you are going to do.
2. **How much** you are going to do.
3. **When** you are going to do it (what time of day).
4. **How many days** a week you are going to do it.

For example: This week I will walk *(what)* around the block *(how much)* before lunch *(when)* three times *(how many)*.

This week I will _____ *(what)*

_____ *(how much)*

_____ *(when)*

_____ *(how many days)*

How certain are you? (circle)   0   1   2   3   4   5   6   7   8   9   1 0

                      not at   totally

                  all certain   certain

For each day you
accomplish your
contract, put a checkmark: Comments

Monday _____   _____

Tuesday _____   _____

Wednesday _____   _____

Thursday _____   _____

Friday _____   _____

Saturday _____   _____

Sunday _____   _____

▼ ▼ ▼ ▼ ▼ ▼ ▼ ▼ ▼ ▼ ▼

PART THREE

Hints, Tips, and Gadgets

▼ ▼ ▼ ▼ ▼ ▼ ▼

8. *Outsmarting Arthritis*

PAIN, FATIGUE, AND STIFFNESS

*P*AIN, fatigue, and stiffness are effects of arthritis that can limit you in a variety of ways. They may prevent you from completing a specific task, hinder the progress of your daily activities, or even leave you feeling completely overwhelmed. From simple physical tasks—unlocking doors, opening jars, getting on buses—to social activities, arthritis can interfere with your life. For example, you may find yourself avoiding new places because you do not know if there will be an accessible bathroom; fear of fatigue may prevent you from entertaining.

As you will discover in this book, exercise, pain-management techniques, and medications can help to alleviate the symptoms of arthritis. In this chapter you will find a number of problem-solving approaches for overcoming various obstacles you may encounter in everyday life. Included are strategies for using your joints appropriately and labor-saving ideas and products that can make your daily activities easier and more pleasant. But before discussing strategies for outsmarting arthritis, it might help to talk more about pain, fatigue, and stiffness.

Pain

As you have learned, for the person with arthritis, pain can occur for different reasons. Performing a stressful activity for *long* periods of time will increase the likelihood of pain. For example, writing a letter for five minutes may cause stress in the fingers but no pain. Continuing to write for an hour might cause pain that lasts for two or three days. Increasing the load on joints will also increase the likelihood of pain. Excess body weight, carrying heavy loads such as grocery bags, climbing stairs, and getting up from a chair are all potentially stressful activities.

Fatigue

Fatigue is a common human experience. It occurs when certain basic needs are not met, for example, not getting proper food, enough sleep, or enough exercise. It can result from inflamed joints or from depression.

Too much activity also causes fatigue. What is too much? For some people, running five miles (8 km) a day is not enough to tire them out, but for others, doing three loads of laundry, standing on the bus during rush hour, or climbing a full flight of stairs may cause fatigue. It's important to know your limits and work within them. In this way, they will gradually become less restricting. Knowing limits is crucial for someone with arthritis. For example, you must be particularly careful not to overdo it when you're beginning to feel good again after an episode of pain. This can cause fatigue or more pain. If you feel fatigued often, consider your diet (see Chapter 14) and your sleeping habits (see Chapter 16), and make sure you are getting enough, but not too much, exercise (see Chapter 10). Also, consider the possibility you may be depressed (see Chapter 17).

Stiffness

Stiffness often occurs when joints are maintained in one position for a long period of time. It is common to experience stiffness in your knees with prolonged sitting. Pain can also aggravate stiffness. The natural reaction to manage a painful joint is to keep it bent or immobile. While this might offer temporary relief, in the long run, it will increase stiffness and may even cause a permanent decrease in joint motion. The final result can be a joint that will not fully bend or straighten. Regular flexibility exercises typically help in maintaining available joint motion over time. Performing flexibility exercises when in one position over a prolonged period can often minimize stiffness, e.g., straightening your knees periodically when you are sitting through a movie.

Pain, fatigue, and stiffness may occur separately or in combination. They can be aggravated if you are so protective of your joints that you avoid all activity. They can also be aggravated if you proceed with an activity as planned and ignore pain, stiffness, or fatigue until they are unbearable. Both ignoring problems and overprotecting joints can lead to a cycle in which pain, fatigue, and stiffness increase. Most likely, this will result in decreased activity levels and increased pain. A good arthritis self-manager will be able to keep them all in check.

Now that you know about pain, fatigue, and stiffness, the next step is to identify how they affect your daily activities.

Steps to Disability

PROBLEM-SOLVING METHOD

Many of the problems caused by arthritis can be solved with the eight-step plan: *identify, pinpoint, list, select, assess, substitute, utilize resources,* and *accept.*

1. **Identify the source of difficulty.** This is the most important step and is probably the most difficult. This step needs to be broken down to help you zero in on the true source of the problem. Identify specific activities that cause you pain, stiffness, or fatigue. If you are having trouble identifying activities that cause problems, review the past twenty-four hours, using the following method:

   ▼ List your activities. Ask yourself if this is more or less activity than you usually do in a day.

   ▼ Check off activities that caused pain in the past.

   ▼ Circle new activities.

   ▼ Look at the checked and circled activities. Repeat those you checked off so you can see if you reproduce the symptoms. (Do not overdo the repetition.)

   ▼ Did your activities keep your joints in one position for long periods?

   ▼ If none of the above help you identify the problem, ask yourself: "Are my joints red, hot, and swollen? Could my arthritis be in an active state? Are my basic needs being met? Am I under extra stress or tension? Have I been taking my medication as prescribed?"

2. **Pinpoint the source of the problem.**
   ▼ What part of the activity caused pain or stiffness?
   ▼ When did fatigue begin?
   ▼ Consider stress, the speed at which you worked, and the duration of the task.

   Pinpoint an activity that you would like to do but feel you cannot. Why can't you do the activity? Is it due to decreased motion, pain, fatigue, stiffness, or weakness? Is your participation being limited by a fear of how others will perceive you?

3. **List ideas that might solve your problem.** If you are short of ideas, ask family or friends for suggestions.

4. **Select an idea that you think will work, and try it out.**

5. **Assess the results.** Did you feel that the problem was completely solved or was it a partial solution? If you still have problems, try the next step.

6. **Substitute another idea from your list if the first one did not work.** Continue to substitute until you exhaust all your ideas.

7. **Utilize resources.** If you exhaust your own ideas without solving the problem, use the following resources: health professionals, books, and the Arthritis Foundation and Arthritis Society.

8. **Accept that the problem may not be solved at this time.** Your present investigation may help you solve the problem or modify the activity in the future.

The following sections discuss techniques that will lengthen your list of ideas and provide you with greater ability to select likely solutions. They may also play a role in preventing future problems by showing you how to get the task done with the least amount of effort. In the final section you will find examples of common problems and of ways to solve them using the method described above.

BODY MECHANICS FOR HOME AND OFFICE

The principle of body mechanics is to use your muscles and joints efficiently in order to reduce stress, pain, and fatigue. Proper attention to these principles can solve many potential problems ahead of time.

1. Distribute the Load over Stronger Joint(s) and/or Larger Surface Area

Purposes

▼ To reduce joint stress and prevent joint pain by spreading the weight of objects you are carrying, pushing, or pulling.

▼ To eliminate tight grasping and pinching, since these actions may stress your knuckles or cause hand stiffness. If you notice deformities developing in your hand(s), ask your doctor about consultation with an occupational therapist. A management program can be developed to meet your specific needs.

Examples

▼ Instead of using your fingers, use the palms of your hand, your forearms, or your elbows.

▼ Instead of your arms, use your whole body. Instead of your back, use your legs.

Wrong

Correct

When using spray cans or bottles, push down with the palm of the hand instead of the fingertip.

Close plastic
containers with
your elbow.

Wring out wet
washcloths or
laundry by wrapping
the item over the
faucet and squeezing
excess water out
between the palms
of your hands. An
alternative is to wrap
the item in a thick
towel and let the
towel soak up the
excess moisture.

Spare your hands from difficult-to-open refrigerator doors or cupboards by placing a strap on the handle. To open, simply place your forearm through the strap and pull.

Instead of holding on to the handles of a rolling pin, place hands flat on top and roll beneath your hands.

To wash dishes, there is a scrubber that fits over your hand available in supermarkets and hardware stores. Since you don't need to grasp it, you can keep your fingers in a straightened position.

▼ Use a sponge instead of a dishrag to mop up tables and counters. The water can be squeezed out of the sponge more easily by putting it in the sink and pressing down with your flattened hand.

Wrong

Correct

When pushing up from a chair, keep your hands facing palm down.

Use your hip to close kitchen or dresser drawers.

Use both arms to take down or hang clothes in the closet.

Instead of placing your fingers through the handle, encircle a coffee cup with both hands. Mugs are especially good for this.

Carry your plate back to the kitchen by "scooping" it up with the palms of both hands.

A Word About Walking Sticks

One way to relieve hip or knee pain is to use a cane or walking stick. The handle of the cane should reach your wrist when your hand is at your side. To make the cane more stable, buy a wide rubber tip at any pharmacy. The tip in most canes is too narrow.

To use a cane, put it in the hand *opposite your bad side*. For example, if your left hip hurts, hold your cane in your right hand. When your left foot is forward, your cane should also be forward. By distributing your weight in this way, you relieve some of the pressure on your hip.

Unfortunately, some people are too proud to use a cane. They think it shows weakness or that they are old. Nothing could be further from the truth. Using a cane shows you are smart and confident enough to do what is best for you.

Canes can also be very stylish. Look around and get a lucite cane, a colored cane, or a fancy cane handle. A cane can be dressed up with a scarf or fancy tape. Some of our self-managers have a whole collection of canes, from walking sticks for picnics to black shiny canes with silver handles for formal affairs.

▼ Holding objects close to your body reduces the load. This in turn reduces fatigue and joint stress. Objects feel heavier if held farther away from your body, and lighter when held closer.

When carrying a briefcase, use a shoulder strap and avoid using the handles. Carry a purse on your forearm or use a shoulder bag and avoid clutching in your hand.

2. Avoid Maintaining the Same Joint Position for Prolonged Periods

Purposes

▼ To reduce joint stiffness

▼ To prevent joint contractures

Examples

▼ **Hips and Knees:** Alternate between sitting and standing positions. Although the sitting position is generally recommended to reduce stress on the lower joints and prevent fatigue, it is important to get up and stretch frequently.

Wrong

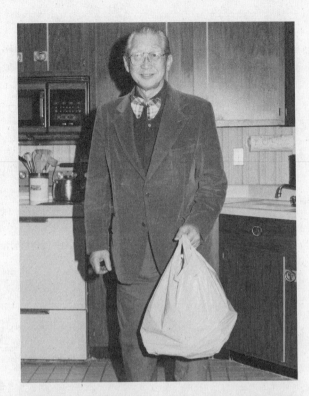

Holding a plastic
grocery bag with
hand down at the
side of the body.

Correct

Holding a brown
paper grocery bag
close to body with
both arms.

▼ **Knees:** When sitting, change the position of your legs so that your knees are periodically stretched out. This can reduce knee stiffness and pain when you return to standing.

▼ **Ankles:** Bend and point your toes while watching television or talking with a friend. You don't have to wait for a specific exercise time to do your stretching exercises (see Chapter 10).

▼ **Hands:** Avoid sustained grasps on objects. For example, instead of writing with a pen, use a typewriter or a computer.

3. Reduce Excess Body Weight

Purpose

▼ To reduce stress on joints and fatigue (see Chapter 14).

4. Use Good Posture

Purpose

A book holder or pillows on your lap serves as a means to support a book and frees your hands.

▼ Proper body alignment when standing, sitting, lifting, and changing positions uses your muscles and joints more efficiently.

Standing

Good posture means that the three curves of your spine, neck, middle back, and lower back are gentle and small. These gentle curves provide stability and absorb shock when you walk and move. Improving your alignment reduces strain on your muscles and joints. Check your posture using the checklist below to identify strengths and weaknesses. Look in a mirror or ask a friend to help you.

▼ Ears directly over your shoulders

▼ Shoulders the same height and relaxed

▼ Shoulders in line with your hips

▼ Stomach muscles lightly contracted

▼ Hips in line with your knees and feet

▼ Knees straight but unlocked

▼ Feet shoulder-width apart

▼ Even weight on both feet

Wrong

Wrong

Correct

Left: Avoid locking your knees, as this puts increased strain on your lower back.

Center: Rounding your shoulders and bringing your head too far forward are common posture mistakes. This position can cause neck and upper-back pain.

Right: Notice that the body is in good alignment. A plumb line dropped from the top of the head will pass through the ear, shoulder, hip, knee, and ankle.

At a computer work station, position your keyboard so that your wrists are in neutral and your elbows are bent at waist height when you type. Select a chair that is comfortable and encourages correct posture. If needed, add a small pillow to support your lower back and a footrest to support your feet.

Place one foot on a footstool. This position helps to reduce back strain during activities that are performed in one position.

Sitting

Position yourself as follows:

- ▼ Head over shoulders.
- ▼ Shoulders relaxed, not elevated (raise your shoulders up to your ears and then relax them to make sure they are not elevated).
- ▼ Upper back straight.
- ▼ Knees even with hips.
- ▼ Buttocks flat on seat.
- ▼ Feet flat on floor or footrest.
- ▼ Even weight on both hips.

Select a chair that:

▼ Has a firm seat.

▼ Has a fairly straight back.

If you are selecting a chair for a work station, choose one that:

▼ Has an adjustable backrest height and angle (avoid chairs with S-shaped curves).

▼ Has an adjustable-height seat so that it is the proper height for your work surface.

▼ Has casters to allow moving from desktop to computer.

▼ Has a rounded end to the seat so that it does not cut into your legs.

When working at your workbench or in the kitchen, a bar-height stool with footrest allows you to half sit, half stand. This helps to prevent fatigue, as well as provide a suitable height for working on projects, washing dishes, or preparing meals.

Standing Up

1. Scoot forward in your chair so that you are near the edge.

2. Place one foot slightly in front of the other so that it is directly under the knee. The other foot is behind the knee.

3. Lean forward until your hips automatically start to come off the chair.

Chairs that are several inches higher than normal, either through the use of pillows or chair leg extenders, make it easier to stand up.

Lifting

Wrong

To lift objects from the ground or low shelves, bend your legs instead of your back: pick up the object, holding it as close to your body as possible, and rise, letting your leg muscles do the work.

People with knee problems may want to let someone else lift heavy objects, since the knees are strained from the weight of the object as well as from their own body weight.

Correct

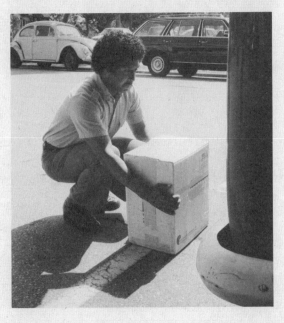

Getting Up from the Floor

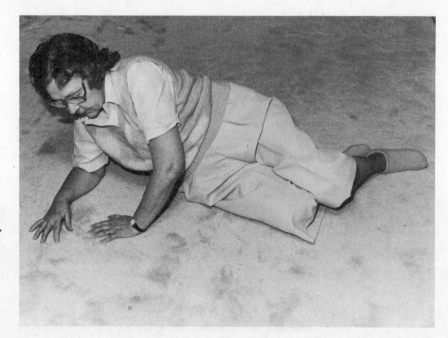

1. Roll onto one side.

2. With the upper hand, push yourself up enough to get your lower elbow under you.

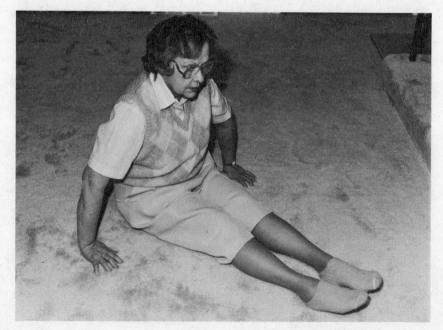

3. Gradually rise until you are sitting up.

4. Reach across your body until both hands are on the floor at one side.

5. *Shift your weight sideways; tuck your knees under and get up onto all fours.*

6. *Crawl to the nearest steady chair and place your hands on the seat for support.*

7. *Putting weight onto your hands, bring one knee up and put that foot flat. Bring your stronger leg into this position, ready to push up.*

8. *Push up with that leg, bearing much of your weight on your hands as they rest on the chair.*

9. When both feet are flat on the floor, begin to straighten your legs. Stop. Keep your head down and let your circulation catch up with the change of positions.

10. Now stand up fully straight. But again, stop a moment before you start to walk. Let your circulation adjust. Many people feel faint if they stand up too fast.

EFFICIENCY PRINCIPLES

If you plan and organize your tasks and workspaces you will eliminate unnecessary steps, which saves time and energy. This helps reduce fatigue. Hasty movements are no more quickly accomplished than organized movements, and they often end in extra work. As the saying goes, "Haste makes waste." Both tension and fatigue are increased when we feel rushed.

1. Plan

Determine the following:

▼ Is the task necessary?

▼ Can the task be simplified?

▼ Who should perform the task?

▼ What steps are involved in completing the task?

▼ In what order will these steps be most efficient?

▼ What is the best time of day or week to perform the task?

▼ Do you need rest periods to complete the task?

▼ What is the best body position to use to complete the task?

Examples

▼ Start large tasks well before the deadline so you can pace yourself, e.g., income tax, school papers, bills, greeting cards.

▼ Make entertaining easier. Spread tasks over several days. Select foods that you can prepare ahead of time. Get help for heavy cleaning.

▼ Alternate repetitive cooking tasks such as cutting, chopping, and stirring to reduce stress on your hands. Take short breaks when cooking large quantities. Alternate sitting and standing to reduce fatigue and joint stress.

▼ Buy vegetables and condiments already chopped in the frozen food and produce section of your grocery to simplify cooking. Salad bars at grocery stores are an excellent place to purchase fresh precut vegetables and fruits.

▼ List your regular cleaning tasks. Create a cleaning schedule that works for you. Consider spreading out light cleaning tasks over a week. Schedule one or two heavy cleaning tasks per month. Complete them on a "good day."

▼ Use computer address and return labels for mail to reduce writing strain.

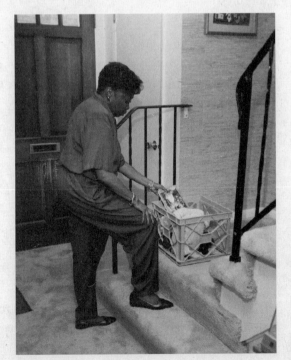

Combine several errands in one trip whenever possible. If you have to go downstairs or to another part of the house or place of work, try to accomplish several things at a time.

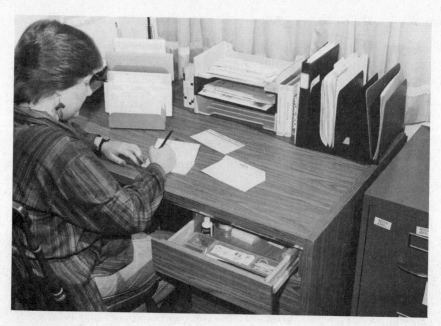

Work on an assembly-line basis. First gather all items you need to complete the task and place them at your workspace. Choose a comfortable position to work, then work in the most efficient order.

2. Organize

Examples

▼ Store equipment and supplies that are regularly used between eye and hip level. This will minimize bending, stooping, and needless searching. Store the heavier items in easy reach, such as on counter-tops.

▼ Use kitchen and office organizers, such as bins, dividers, turntables, and spice racks to locate items quickly.

▼ Store items in the location where they are most frequently used.

▼ Eliminate clutter. Remove unnecessary or infrequently used items from shelves.

▼ To remove clutter: put items you do not use in a bin. If you do not look for these in a month, get rid of them. If you have a very cluttered area, put away one item every time you pass by. Clutter does not have to be organized all at one time.

▼ Put duplicates of inexpensive items such as cleaner, scissors, and cellophane tape in all the places where they are regularly used.

▼ Special organizers are available for closets to maximize your use of space.

▼ Store seasonal items such as winter hats and scarfs in clear plastic containers so they are easy to locate.

Organize storage areas with dividers, special racks, turntables, and pull-out shelves. Many of these items are available in local stores or can be easily made by a carpenter.

*Use pegboards
and hooks to
hang objects.*

3. Balance Work with Rest

One of the most effective means of avoiding fatigue is to schedule short but frequent rest periods throughout the day. Forcing ourselves to rest before we get tired is often difficult. We all want to get our work done. If we can prevent fatigue, even if it means stopping in the middle of a job, our endurance over the long run will be increased. While stopping to rest is difficult, remember that long work periods require longer recovery periods.

Examples

▼ Schedule frequent rest periods throughout the day. These will vary for each individual. An example might be to rest ten minutes out of every hour, instead of working for three hours straight. Even a short break is better than nothing.

▼ Alternate heavy and light work tasks during each day. In addition, plan the more difficult or lengthy tasks when you know you have the endurance to do them.

▼ Sitting to work is a form of rest since it uses less energy than standing. However, if you spend your workday behind a desk, you will find that moving around at regular intervals will help to keep you more alert and energetic.

PRODUCT-SELECTION PRINCIPLES

Using products with the features described in this section helps reduce joint stress, pain, and fatigue by allowing you to complete a task with the least amount of effort. These principles help you choose new products and evaluate those you already own.

If you need information about finding any of these items call your Arthritis Foundation and Arthritis Society chapter or contact the occupational therapy department at your local hospital.

1. Use Wheels

Purposes

▼ To reduce friction, lessening the resistance between surfaces

▼ To avoid lifting and carrying

Examples

▼ Use a cart or attach a carrier with wheels to items to avoid the strain of carrying.

2. Use Extended Handles

Purpose

▼ Products with long handles or long attachments let you use less force to manipulate objects. These products help conserve strength.

Use a luggage carrier or suitcase on wheels when traveling. This allows you to take most of the strain off your arms as you push or pull the suitcase.

Use wheels to transport. Utility carts, tea tables, and shopping carts are just a few examples of readily available items on wheels.

Special key-holders allow you to turn a key by holding the handle in the palm of your hand. These are available through special-equipment firms or can be made by riveting a piece of wood or metal to the key.

Examples

▼ A piece of wood, metal, or firm plastic can be attached to many types of objects to increase the length of the handle.

3. Use Lightweight Objects

Purpose

▼ To reduce joint stress, pain, and fatigue.

Examples

Lightweight objects are easier to carry and to clean. The following chart lists a few examples of lighter weight objects.

LIGHTWEIGHT OPTIONS FOR EVERYDAY OBJECTS

ITEM	LIGHTWEIGHT OPTIONS	WHAT TO AVOID
Dishes	plastic Corelle Heller	stoneware
Pots/pans	Metrolight Prochief Frazier	iron skillet
Bowls	plastic aluminum	Pyrex stoneware
Baking dishes and casseroles	foil pans aluminum microwave cookware Farberware T-fal	Corningware
Luggage/briefcases	nylon canvas	leather hardback
Fans	plastic	metal
Winter coats	fiberfill goose down	leather wool

A doorknob extender allows you to open the door with the palm of the hand instead of with the fingers.

Open a car door with an aid in the palm of your hand.

4. Use Large Handles

Purposes

- ▼ To help maintain a secure hold when hands are weak.
- ▼ To help hold an object if fingers do not fully close.
- ▼ To lessen tension required to maintain your hold on objects.

Examples

- ▼ Purchase silverware, pens, tools, etc. that are made with bulky handles about one inch (2.5 cm) in diameter.

Attach a dowel or a piece of wood to a can opener and hold on to this lengthened handle when opening cans. Never use a butterfly can opener. The pressure required to operate one is extreme; use an electric or wall-mounted type.

Open flip-top cans with a knife.

▼ Pipe-insulation tubing with an opening from 3/8 to 3/4 inch (1 to 2 cm) in diameter offers an easy and inexpensive way to build up utensil handles. You may need to tape the slit in the tubing shut. Most hardware stores sell pipe-insulation tubing in four-foot (1.2 m) lengths at reasonable prices.

▼ Pencil grips may be purchased from office-supply stores or ordered from daily living equipment catalogues.

5. Use Convenience Items

Purposes

▼ To decrease the length of time and number of steps needed to complete a task
▼ To reduce joint stress and pain and fatigue

Examples

▼ Use labor-saving devices such as a food processor, blender, microwave, electric toothbrush, and electric hedger.
▼ Purchase permanent press clothing.

Foam padding added to such articles as a toothbrush, pen, razor, fork, and comb increases the size of the handle.

Pencil grip

PUTTING IT ALL TOGETHER

Now you have all the information you need to apply the eight-step problem-solving method to some of the problems interfering with your daily routine. Here are some examples of how the problem-solving method is used. It is important to note that the solution to the problem varies from case to case, depending on the situation surrounding the problem. It won't always be necessary to go through all eight steps.

Example 1

Identify:	I can't open jars.
Pinpoint:	It sometimes causes pain; I'm too weak.
List Ideas:	Ask spouse or neighbor.
	Use cans and open with electric can opener.
	Buy commercial jar opener.

Use sheet of rubber to produce more friction by placing over lid.

Release suction with a knife.

Tap jar upside down.

Select: Tried to release suction.

Assess: Worked on some jars but not others.

Substitute: Buy commercial jar opener.

Assess: It's wonderful!

Example 2

Identify: My joints are red, hot, and swollen. Activities seem to make them worse. My doctor says to rest and do what I can.

List Ideas: Stay in bed.

Keep up my regular routine.

Meet basic needs by getting sufficient sleep, eat well, reduce tension as much as possible, and exercise appropriately.

Decrease activities that can wait.

Delegate tasks, modify tasks.

Select: Stay in bed.

Assess: Stayed in bed and did not move for two days. I feel less fatigue, but my joints are stiff. I think I lost strength.

Substitute: Try three ideas at once: meet basic needs, decrease activities that can wait, and delegate tasks or modify tasks.

Assess: I feel better. In order to reduce tension, I stopped all activities that can wait, and delegated tasks to family and friends. I move my joints twice a day and feel less stiff. I still shower and dress daily. Note: This period of active arthritis seemed milder than usual.

Example 3

Identify: I can't go on vacation.

Pinpoint: I can't walk long distances in airports. How will I find accessible bathrooms?

List Ideas: Bring raised toilet seat.

Call hotel in advance regarding bathrooms.

Call travel agent.

Contact airlines regarding wheelchair.

Select: Call travel agent.

Assess: Travel agent booked me on an airline with wheelchair service from cab to plane. She contacted the hotel and investigated bathroom status. I still need to bring my raised toilet seat.

Example 4

Identify: My body aches after working at my desk for an hour.

Pinpoint: Suspect desk is too high.

List Ideas: Elevate chair by adding cushion.
Work at different location with a lower table.
Purchase new chair.

Select: Add cushion.

Assess: The cushion improved the work height but now my feet are off the floor. I added a small block under my feet, which helped tremendously.

Example 5

Identify: I have joint pain during intercourse.

List Ideas: Grin and bear it.
Make up excuses to avoid.
Find resources to learn new positions, i.e., call Arthritis Foundation.
Discuss with mate.

Select: Grin and bear it.

Assess: Pain increased and now I am making excuses. My spouse seems frustrated.

Substitute: Call Arthritis Foundation; ask for names of resources.

Assess: Received a copy of *Living and Loving*. Tried suggestions in the book and my spouse noticed the difference. I admitted my pain and we are reviewing other resources together.

Example 6

Identify: I am afraid to visit friends for brunch. How will I use the toilet?

List Ideas: Stay home.
Bring raised toilet seat.
Call friend and ask about her toilet accessibility.
Use toilet before leaving, bring raised toilet seat but leave in car.

Select: Call friend and ask about toilet height.

Assess: Friend suggested I come early and bring toilet seat before other guests arrive to avoid embarrassment. She will store it in the bathroom closet.

Example 7

Identify: My knees feel stiff and sore after sitting in a movie theater.

List Ideas: Walk to lobby once an hour.
Sit in aisle seat and stretch legs every fifteen minutes.
Sit in last row and stand when I need to.

Select: Walk to lobby once an hour.

Assess: This wasn't enough to decrease stiffness. I felt embarrassed to get up more than that.

Substitute: Sit in aisle seat and stretch legs every fifteen minutes.

Assess: This helped, but I decided every ten minutes worked better for me.

Example 8

Identify: I have trouble unlocking doors.

Pinpoint: My fingers are too weak to turn keys. Repeated attempts hurt my fingers.

List Ideas: Oil lock.
Lengthen area to grasp—add handle extension.
Ask in hardware store if larger keys are available.

Select: Add handle extension.

Assess: Attached key to piece of plastic with wire. I can open the door on the first or second attempt.

Example 9

Identify: I'm exhausted when I carry groceries. Sometimes my back hurts.

List Ideas: Carry smaller loads.
Hold groceries closer to body.
Seek assistance: Ask family or friend, pay to have groceries delivered.
Use pelvic tilt when carrying groceries.
Use cart or wagon.
Use backpack.

Select: Seek assistance.

Assess: Worked well first time, but my friend seemed to resent the request in the third consecutive week and refused.

Substitute: Carry smaller loads and hold close to body.

Assess: Able to manage one bag half filled. Contacted friend and asked for help once a month. She said yes. Combining both ideas seems to work well.

▼ ▼ ▼ ▼ ▼ ▼ ▼

9. Self-Helpers: 100+ Hints and Aids

The preceding chapter, "Outsmarting Arthritis," provided you with basic principles and examples of how to use your joints appropriately. Additional hints are provided in this chapter, not only on how to use your joints, but also on how to perform activities if your general mobility or finger coordination is impaired.

You may find that you are already doing many of the things mentioned in this chapter. It is true that necessity is the mother of invention. If you combine your needs and your common sense, you will probably come up with another hundred hints. Use the suggestions here as a springboard for additional ideas for making your life easier and more comfortable. Then share them with friends and others who might benefit from them.

DRESSING

If buttons are difficult to manipulate, sew Velcro on clothing. Attach buttons permanently to the top side, and use the Velcro as a fastener. Velcro can be found in most sewing stores.

An alternative to buttons on sleeves is elasticized thread sewn on button cuffs. This often provides sufficient give for your hands to slide through.

In the future, buy clothes that are easy to put on and easy to care for. Tops should be large enough or designed so that sleeves are easy to slip into—you may want to avoid turtlenecks. Elastic waistbands around pants should be loose enough to slip easily over hips. Fastenings should be located in the front and be easy to manipulate.

If reaching the clothes in the closet is difficult, have someone lower the rod.

Special devices to assist with shoes include long-handled shoe horns, elastic shoelaces, and zipper laces. Velcro can be useful for fastening shoes as well as clothing.

Buttonhooks work well to fasten buttons. You can make your own buttonhook with a six inch (15 cm) piece of wooden dowel and a large paper clip.

A bent coat hanger, reacher, or dressing stick can assist with pulling pants up, straightening shirts, or retrieving clothes slightly out of reach.

Place large rings, thread, or leather hoops on zipper tabs.

Fasten your bra in front of you. Turn bra around and pull it into place. Try front-closure bras.

Shoes

When buying shoes, look for the following features:

▼ Low heel, no higher than one inch (2.5 cm).
▼ Toe area wide and deep enough to prevent rubbing or crunching of toes.
▼ Cushion sole to pad the ball of your foot; avoid wooden soles.
▼ Laces, buckles, or Velcro to loosen or tighten when feet swell.
▼ Soft upper material to give or be stretched to relieve pressure on specific areas.

Don't rule out gym shoes. Many running and aerobic shoes meet the above criteria. Some now have Velcro closures. If your present shoes have the recommended characteristics but are still uncomfortable, consult your physician or podiatrist.

There are a variety of shoe adaptations available, such as the following:

▼ Gel soles
▼ Soft cushion inserts
▼ Custom-molded inserts
▼ Pads for ball of foot
▼ External bar under shoe

A sock aid will allow you to put on your socks if you cannot reach your feet. First, you need to slide your sock onto the sock aid shell. Then drop the sock aid to the floor. Slide your foot into the shell and pull the sock on gently with the long handles. You can make your own sock aid (right) by cutting x-ray film or construction board into the shape of a "ten gallon hat" and attaching a piece of cord through a hole punched in each side of the "hat's brim."

Most of them take pressure off the ball of the foot. Consult your physician or podiatrist when choosing the proper adaptation for you. Foot problems are very individual.

BATHING AND HYGIENE

A long-handled sponge or brush can be used to soap yourself when bathing.

Tub and shower benches, or a webbed plastic lawn chair, allow you to sit while showering. This helps prevent fatigue and provides a place to sit when getting down into the tub is difficult.

Safety considerations when bathing include the use of nonskid safety strips or a rubber bathmat on the floor. In addition, grab bars can be permanently installed on the wall or attached to the edge of the bathtub. Grab bars provide a safe hold when you are climbing in and out of the tub or shower and also provide a place to pull or push up from when you are in the tub.

A long shower spray hose makes rinsing easier.

After bathing, put on a terry robe and let it soak up the water as you pat yourself dry. This lets you avoid the sometimes painful motions needed to towel yourself dry.

Use a shower caddy to keep soap and shampoo within easy reach.

Special long-handled combs and brushes are useful when shoulder and elbow limitations prevent you from reaching your head.

In addition, a toilet safety frame or a grab bar installed in the wall next to the toilet will allow you to use your arms when sitting and standing.

Electric toothbrushes and Water-Piks make oral hygiene easier. In addition, there is a device that holds dental floss, allowing you to floss your teeth with one hand holding onto the handle—ask your dentist about these or check your local drugstore.

Put foam curlers onto eyeliner and mascara handles for better grip.

Use the heel of your hand to squeeze the toothpaste tube or press down on a toothpaste pump.

The Freshette Director makes it possible for women to urinate while standing. It is a part of a complete portable restroom system that can be used standing, sitting in a chair, or lying in bed.

A bath mitt can be bought or easily made by sewing two facecloths together. Lather it up and soap yourself the easy way.

A raised toilet seat or commode over the toilet provides greater height and thus makes standing up easier.

For feminine hygiene, wind tampon string around a pencil. Keep pencil horizontal and pull gently with both hands for easier removal. Some brands of tampons have loops rather than straight strings, with which you can more easily use a pencil or your fingers to pull. For those who use pads, a detachable shower hose with an adjustable spray may be useful for more thorough genital-area cleaning.

Enlarge the handle of a razor by adding utensil foam pipe insulation or tubing or by taping a small sponge around the handle.

Ask family members to fold the end of the toilet paper into a V. This makes the paper easier to grasp.

COOKING

Microwave ovens save time and energy. They are easy to operate, easy to clean, and usually easy to reach since they are often placed on countertops.

To avoid lifting pots heavy with food and the water the food was boiled in, consider several alternatives. One is to place a frying basket inside a pot so you can lift the food out with the basket and drain the water later. Spaghetti cookers come with a perforated insert and can serve in the same manner. Or you may want to ladle the contents out.

To open jars, install a jar opener that will grip the lid as you use both hands to turn the jar itself. Also, ask other members of the family not to close lids too tightly.

Use lightweight cooking utensils, bowls, and dishes. Avoid cast-iron skillets and heavy ceramic bowls.

Select appliances with levers or push buttons that are easy to operate.

Store canned goods so that the same items are lined up behind one another. This way you can tell from the front label what is in the back of the shelf.

Plan and prepare meals ahead of time to avoid last-minute preparations. Cook some meals the day before, and then heat them up again the next day. Also, try preparing double or triple portions and freezing the extra.

Find dishes that require minimal preparation and little effort. Today many convenience foods, ready mixes, and frozen foods contain low salt, low fat, and minimal additives.

One-pot meals require less cleanup.

Serve foods in the same containers in which they were cooked. Use casseroles, Farberware, and other lightweight attractive cooking vessels.

Use throw-away pie tins and other disposable utensils. This cuts down on dishwashing.

Line pans with aluminum foil to make cleanup easier.

Use cookie tins and pans with special surfaces that prevent sticking and messy cleanup, or spray them with a nonstick product.

You can cut with your wrist in a neutral position using an ergonomic knife or a pizza cutter. They are available in a variety of sizes and styles.

Opener for soda and beer cans

Jar opener

When peeling vegetables, try the kind of peeler with a handle you can slip your fingers through, or build up the handle of a standard peeler.

Use a pot with a wet cloth draped over it as a support for a bowl when pouring batter into a baking pan.

The "T" Turning Handle makes it easier to turn the knobs on stoves and washing machines.

Mixing bowls can be stabilized by placing them on a wet washcloth or on little octopus-like suction cups. You can also place the bowl in a drawer at work height.

Place flour and sugar in containers so you can scoop out the amount needed and avoid lifting heavy bags each time.

Mitt pot holders allow you to lift hot pans with the palms of both hands.

Use a bent coat hanger or dowel with a hook to pull oven shelves out when checking on the meal.

Attach a spray hose at the kitchen sink so that you can fill pots with water on the countertop; slide pots to the stove to avoid lifting.

If you cannot afford an electric food processor use an onion chopper or a Femster.

Try using a pizza wheel instead of a knife to cut various foods.

Food processors make food preparation a snap, especially when large quantities of food must be chopped, sliced, or grated.

ENTERTAINING

Arrange a buffet meal. Let your guests select their own silver, plates, and napkins and serve themselves from large dishes of food.

Use nice paper plates and plastic utensils to eliminate dishwashing.

Have a potluck meal, where each guest brings a dish of food or some paper goods.

HOUSEKEEPING

Keep a set of cleaning supplies in each area where they are used, to eliminate needless walking.

To clean the bathtub, sit on a low stool next to the tub and use a long-handled sponge.

Long-handled sponges can also be used to clean around door sills and other hard-to-reach places.

Use a long-handled dustpan and small broom to clean up dry spills from floors.

Use an adjustable-height ironing board so that you can sit to iron. Attach a cord-minder to keep the cord out of your way.

Carpeting or foam-backed rugs help to ease ankle and foot pain when prolonged standing and moving about are necessary.

Use gravity whenever possible. Let your clothes fall from the dryer into the basket. When scooping them out, you may want to use a reacher or stick.

Laundry bags that were originally intended for washing delicate items like nylons can be used for all small pieces of clothing (socks, underwear) and thus eliminate searching in the machine.

If lifting a heavy detergent box is difficult, you can either have someone else pour some into a smaller container or scoop it out. Liquid detergents may also be more manageable.

Use a back-preserver tool on your floor mop or push broom. Tasks can be performed with better posture and less strain to the back with this special long-handled attachment.

Enlarged knobs are available to place on lamps as well as appliances such as washing machines (certain brands only) to increase ease of handling. Check with your washing machine manufacturer if the controls are difficult to operate.

Try using the old-style push-on clothespins rather than pinch clothespins.

Front-loading washers are generally easier to use than top-loading washers. Raising the washer on blocks will also make laundering easier, since bending is eliminated.

Call your local grocery to find out whether they deliver at an affordable price. Sometimes a local teenager can shop for you more economically. Also, senior centers often offer shopping services.

Use lockable casters on furniture. It will be easier to move when cleaning. These allow you to roll the furniture when you wish but they lock in place for everyday use.

Use a large spatula or an oven shovel to tuck in sheets.

The Touch-tronic, a device that fits into the light socket, allows you to turn lamps on and off by touching them with your fingers. It can be ordered from lighting stores.

WORK

At a computer work station:

▼ Use a keyboard that is detachable from the screen. Avoid prolonged use of laptop computers as they encourage poor head and neck posture.

▼ Add a small towel roll behind your lower back if your chair does not provide sufficient support.

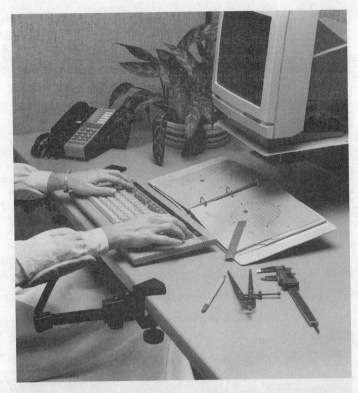

Forearm supports move with you as you work at a computer terminal. They reduce strain in the arms, neck, and shoulders by providing additional support. Consider these if you are unable to work at a conventional computer work station.

This angled work surface encourages good posture during reading and writing tasks. It reduces strain on the neck and upper back.

▼ Select a document holder that is the same height and distance from you as your screen.

▼ Position your monitor so that the upper third of the screen is level with your eyes.

▼ Use a footrest if your feet do not touch the floor.

▼ Consider forearm supports or wrist rests if your chair does not have supportive arms.

▼ Position your arms so that your elbows form a 90-degree angle.

▼ Keep your elbow and wrist in a neutral position parallel to the floor.

▼ Consider getting head phones if you use the phone while you type or write.

When writing at a desk, do not lean forward; sit tall and bend the neck only slightly. People with neck problems may want to consider getting a drafting table with an adjustable slant.

Take a break from prolonged sitting, and do exercises to reduce tension, such as Shoulder Rolls, (page 127), Two-way Neck Stretch (page 124), or Hi and Bye (page 129).

If you build up the handle on a conventional leash (left), you can use a less forceful grip. If your dog likes to sniff or roam, consider a Flexi-Leash (right), which expands and retracts with your dog's movement. The flexibility of this leash can reduce strain on your back and arm.

RECREATION OR LEISURE TIME

An embroidery frame that can be attached to a table or chair will allow you to do needlework and sewing without using your hands to stabilize the article. These are available primarily through self-help aid catalogs.

If you like to play cards, try using a card holder. These can be purchased through mail-order catalogs or easily made by sawing a slit in a piece of wood. You can also make your own card holder with a box. Simply take the cover off and put it under the box. Your cards can be lined up in the lip of the lid and rest against the box.

Afternoon exercises or sports are a really good way to break up the day. Try to set up a schedule to work where you can take an extended break to swim or exercise during the lunch hour.

When gardening, try sitting on a small stool instead of kneeling to weed or plant. If you prefer kneeling, consider knee pads or the Easy Kneeler.

Gardening can be made even easier by having planter boxes or raised flower beds made. This eliminates stooping entirely, as you can sit to work at a comfortable level.

If you enjoy gardening, there is now an attachment for shovels and a different attachment to be used with hoes and rakes. These back-preserver tools can easily be attached to your own equipment.

The Easy Kneeler allows you to lower yourself down and push yourself up with minimal strain. It also can be turned over and used as a seat to work in raised flower beds or planter boxes.

If threading a needle is difficult, self-threading needles or automatic threading machines are available through catalogs and in some sewing stores.

Use loop scissors when sewing to avoid pressure and pain on the thumb joint.

Rolling scissors reduce hand strain. They roll along the cutting surface.

You can make any tool more ergonomic by attaching this clamp-on pistol grip. It helps to keep the wrist in a neutral position while you are working.

DRIVING

When buying a car, look for doors that are easy to open and close, storage that is easy to reach, such as in a hatchback model, and a seat positioner that is easy to manipulate.

Attach a loop of fabric to the inside door handle to make it easier to close. (See photo of loop on refrigerator door, page 55.)

Auxiliary or wide-angle mirrors allow for increased visibility when neck movement is limited.

To make driving more comfortable and prevent back strain, look into obtaining cushions for the car. You can purchase cushions that are positioned on the upright portion of the seat or those you can sit on to improve posture and prevent slouching. Many cars now come equipped with a lumbar support for the driver. If you use this support, make sure it does not push your back so far forward that it is painful.

KEEPING JOINTS WARM

Use the extra-long heating pads that wrap around an arm or leg and fasten with Velcro to warm an elbow or knee.

Soak stiff, sore, or cold hands in warm water. This is especially useful to loosen them from morning stiffness. At night, warm the hands in this manner; rub hand lotion in and wear cotton gloves while sleeping.

Thermoelastic gloves are especially warming, since they are made from wool and elastic fibers. They are available in some pharmacies.

Thermoelastic products are also available for knees and elbows. A soft, thick knee sock should also be used in the same manner. Cut the sock so you have a tube approximately seven inches (18 cm) long and place the tube over your knee or elbow. Microwavable heat wraps are available for the hand, wrist, knee, elbow, ankle, and torso.

Use electric blankets as a lightweight cover; they are especially useful in warming the bed before you get in it.

An alternative way to stay warm during the night or when resting is to sleep inside a sleeping bag that is placed under a blanket. The bag will turn with you and prevent cold air spaces.

Use a sleeping bag, cozy-wrap, or comforter when reading in a chair.

Use a mug to drink hot tea or coffee and hold it between both hands to warm them.

Slipper socks, worn over a pair of regular socks, will help to keep feet and ankles warm.

A foot bath not only will warm your feet as they soak in the water but also can act as a massager.

Dress warmly. Use long underwear even in the spring and fall.

Place a space heater or heat lamp in your bathroom and turn it on before showering in the morning.

Stand by the radiator to warm up, or build a fire in the fireplace.

COMFORT

When sitting for long periods of time is necessary, such as when riding in a car or flying, you can relax your back muscles by doing the following: Place your forearms on your thighs, hands near the knees, and lean forward with your face as near to the knees as possible. Breathe deeply and relax in this position. Come up to sitting slowly. Repeat several times.

Purchase a padded toilet seat, or sew a cover for it out of thick furry material.

Pad chairs with pillows or foam cushions.

If you don't want to take a pillow with you when you go out, take a sweater or jacket along to use as a cushion for hard chairs.

Recliner chairs with head supports are comfortable for many people, especially those with neck problems.

Electric beds are no longer confined to the hospital. Home models are available that have movable back and foot sections.

Be sure that you have adequate lighting and ventilation for all activities.

If you take aspirin for pain, you may want to wake up early, take your aspirin, and go back to sleep until it begins to work. Keep aspirin and a glass of water at the bedside.

Splints, often made for hands from special plastics, help to maintain proper joint alignment, prevent stress, and reduce pain. Your physician can refer you to an occupational therapist who can construct one for you.

An Ace bandage can also provide some added stability to joints, as well as serve as a reminder to use them appropriately.

MISCELLANEOUS

To control lamps, equipment, and appliances in inaccessible locations, there is a plug on the market with an on-off switch. This can be plugged in directly to a wall outlet or can be attached to an extension cord that can be positioned near you.

An easier, though quite expensive, method of controlling appliances and lights is with a Home Control Unit. Available through certain large department stores, this device consists of a command console and up to sixteen module units for each appliance wanted. Pushing the buttons on the console will turn any appliance on or off anywhere in your house.

Use a clipboard to keep writing paper steady.

A felt-tip pen allows you to write with less pressure.

Mechanical reachers extend your reach by two to three feet (60 to 90 cm), allowing you to retrieve items from the floor or high shelves.

When attending lectures, use a cassette recorder to eliminate hurried note taking.

When shaking hands with another person, grasp the fingers or wrist of the person's hands first so that his or her thumb cannot grasp and squeeze your hand too hard.

Use a steak or paring knife at dinner, since the sharper the knife, the less pressure is needed. Be careful.

Make sure the chairs you use at home are easy to get out of—if not, you may not want to get out of them often enough to move around and loosen up. Avoid soft, low chairs.

PURCHASING "ADAPTIVE EQUIPMENT" FROM MEDICAL AND SELF-HELP CATALOGUES

Today a number of companies specialize in equipment for people with physical limitations. At the end of this chapter, there is a listing of several companies that sell equipment to the public through mail order catalogues. When you are choosing equipment for yourself, be selective. Identify specific tasks that interfere with your independence on a regular basis and look for equipment that is likely to make these tasks easier. For example, if opening your front door or starting your car causes hand pain, a key extender might reduce your pain. On the other hand, if holding your silverware is difficult for you, consider building up the handles with pipe insulation tubing or buying utensils with broader handles in your local department or discount stores before shopping in catalogues. Adaptive equipment can make tasks easier and even pain-free. Sometimes homemade adaptive equipment or modifying the way you do the activity can achieve the same goal.

Sources for Equipment

Many items described in Chapters 8 and 9 are available in local department stores, hardware stores, gardening shops, or discount chain stores. You can also consider making your own adaptive aids with inexpensive supplies. Should you decide to purchase adaptive aids, some are available at medical supply stores in your area or from the companies listed below, which sell to the general public through the mail. (For equipment resources outside the United States, contact the arthritis organization in your country.)

GARDENING SUPPLIES

Gardener's Supply
128 Intervale Rd.
Burlington, VT 05401
Phone: 802-863-1700
      800-955-3370
Fax: 802-660-4600

Walt Nicke Co.
36 McCleod Lane
P.O. Box 433
Topsfield, MA 01983
Phone: 508-887-3388
      800-822-4114
Fax: 508-774-6584

SEATING AND DESK EQUIPMENT

The BackCare Corporation
200 S. Desplaines
Chicago, IL 60661
Phone: 312-258-0888
Fax: 312-258-0090

Ergonomic Solutions
129 N. Sylvan Drive
Mundelein, IL 60060-3307
Phone: 708-566-4949
Fax: 708-566-7235

Ergo Source
4250 Norex Drive
Chaska, MN 55318-3047
Phone: 800-969-4374
Fax: 800-375-1119

Ergonomic Technology
135 Carlisle Rd.
Deerfield, IL 60015
Phone: 708-945-0009
Fax: 708-945-0042

DAILY LIVING EQUIPMENT

Activities for Daily Living
Smith and Nephew Rolyan
P.O. Box 1005
Germantown, WI 53022
Phone: 800-545-7758
Fax: 800-545-7758
Fax: 414-251-7758

After Therapy Catalog
NCM Consumer Products Division
P.O. Box 6070
San Jose, CA 95150-6070
Phone: 800-235-7054
Fax: 408-277-6824

Aids for Arthritis, Inc.
3 Little Knoll Court
Medford, NJ 08055
Phone: 609-654-6918

Enrichments
P.O. Box 471
Western Springs, IL 60558
Phone: 800-323-5547
Fax: 800-547-4333
Fax: 708-325-4602

Freshette
D.M.S.
1554 Agnew Street
Simi Valley, CA 93065
Phone: 805-527-1244
Fax: 805-527-1244

Sears Home Healthcare
P.O. Box 19009
Provo, UT 84604
Phone: 800-326-1750
Fax: 800-278-8808

Vandenberg
16706 S. Oak Park Ave.
Tinley Park, IL 60477
Phone: 800-872-2347
Fax: 708-532-2676

▼ ▼ ▼ ▼ ▼ ▼ ▼ ▼ ▼ ▼ ▼

PART FOUR

Keeping Your Body Healthy

10. Exercise for Fitness

THE SPIRIT of exercise and fitness is everywhere. Well, almost everywhere. It's easy to see why arthritis and an active life can be hard to combine. When you want to exercise but aren't sure what to do, arthritis pain, stiffness, and the fear of doing harm can be powerful forces to overcome. Until recently, many people with arthritis knew they should "exercise for arthritis"; however, they thought exercising for fun and fitness was only for others.

New information has changed how we think about exercise and arthritis. Thanks to many people with arthritis who have volunteered to exercise in research studies, we can now advise exercise for fun and fitness for people with arthritis. A regular exercise program that includes flexibility, strengthening, and aerobic exercises lessens fatigue, builds stronger muscles and bones, increases your flexibility, gives you more stamina, and improves your general health and sense of well-being—all important for good arthritis care. People with arthritis have improved fitness with exercise that includes walking, bicycling, or aquatic exercise. After two or three months most exercisers also reported less pain, anxiety, and depression.

Traditional medical care of arthritis is based on helping people mainly when their arthritis flares. During a flare it's important to rest more and to protect the inflamed joints. But continuing to be inactive after the flare is over can be bad for your health and actually increase some arthritis problems. Unused joints, bones, and muscles deteriorate quickly. Long periods of inactivity can lead to weakness, stiffness, fatigue, poor appetite, constipation, high blood pressure, obesity, osteoporosis, and increased sensitivity to pain, anxiety, and depression. These are some of the same problems that occur when a person has arthritis. So it can become difficult to tell whether it is arthritis, inactivity, or some combination of the two that is to blame.

In this chapter you will learn about physical fitness and the different types of fitness exercises so you will be able to make wise exercise choices.

This advice is not intended to take the place of therapeutic exercises. If you've had an exercise plan prescribed for you or have any questions, take this book to your doctor or therapist and ask what he or she thinks about this program.

WHAT IS PHYSICAL FITNESS?

Physical fitness for people is much like good maintenance and proper use for an automobile. Both allow you to start when you want, enjoy a smooth and relaxed trip, get to your destination without a breakdown, and have some fuel in your tank when you arrive. How well an automobile works depends on its points and plugs, filters, hoses, tires, lubrication, and fuel systems. Physical fitness for humans is a combination of the following:

▼ Cardiovascular fitness (heart, lungs, and blood vessels)
▼ Muscle strength
▼ Muscle endurance
▼ Flexibility
▼ Percent of body fat

A regular exercise program that includes flexibility, strengthening, and aerobic activities will improve and maintain physical fitness.

Fitness is possible for people of all abilities, sizes, shapes, ages, and attitudes. Just as looking at a parked automobile doesn't tell you much about how it drives, appearance won't tell you much about a person's physical fitness. That new, shiny model may not perform as well as the well-maintained car that has a few dents or a little rust. There is another important similarity between keeping your body fit and your car running: Both work best when used regularly and responsibly.

Regular exercise benefits everyone. By exercising you can reduce your risk for diabetes, cardiovascular disease, and osteoporosis. You increase your stamina and have more energy. Regular exercise helps control weight and avoid constipation. When you exercise, you feel better about yourself and your abilities.

PHYSICAL FITNESS AND ARTHRITIS

If you have arthritis, regular exercise and fitness have special benefits.

1. Strong muscles that do not tire quickly help protect joints by improving stability and absorbing shock.

2. Good flexibility lessens pain and reduces the risk of sprains and strains.

3. Maintaining a good weight helps take stress off weight-bearing joints.

4. Regular exercise helps nourish joints and keeps cartilage and bone healthy.

5. Higher energy levels, less anxiety and depression, and less discomfort are other advantages to exercise and fitness.

Thinking of your exercise as a physical fitness program helps you take a positive, mainstream approach to exercise. By understanding physical fitness and exercise, you'll be able to improve your health, feel better, and manage your arthritis, too. Feeling more in control and less at the mercy of arthritis is one of the greatest benefits of becoming an exercise self-manager.

YOUR OWN FITNESS PROGRAM

An exercise program to improve physical fitness includes exercises for flexibility, strength, endurance, and cardiovascular fitness. How you choose to combine these different types of exercise depends on your current abilities, exercise experience, and the goals you want to accomplish.

To be a successful exercise self-manager, you need to understand what the different types of exercise can do for you and how to use them to meet your goals. The following section introduces you to the three basic types of exercise: flexibility, strengthening, and aerobic exercise. The "Fitness Exercises" table on page 108 is a quick exercise reference. Details and instructions for doing the exercises are in Chapters 11, 12, and 13.

Flexibility Exercises

Flexibility exercises, also known as range-of-motion and stretching exercises, are the foundation of any exercise program. They are especially important for the person with arthritis. The purpose is to increase or maintain flexibility and motion in muscles, tendons, ligaments, and joints. Flexibility is necessary for comfortable movement during exercise and daily activities, and to reduce the risk of sprains and strains. Flexibility is also important for good posture and strength.

Flexibility exercises are done gently and smoothly, three to ten times each, usually every day. Flexibility exercises should also be performed before any more vigorous type of exercise.

If you haven't exercised regularly in some time, or have pain, stiffness, or weakness that interferes with your daily activities, begin your fitness program

FITNESS EXERCISES: QUICK-REFERENCE GUIDE

TYPE	SUGGESTIONS FOR USE	BENEFITS
Flexibility	Daily routine	Flexibility
	Get in shape for strengthening/aerobics	Comfort
		Joint health
	Aerobics warm-up	Easier daily activity
	As needed for comfort	Relaxation
Strength	Every-other-day routine	Protect joints
	With flexibility exercise	Easier daily activity
	With flexibility and aerobic for total fitness program	Relieve pain
		Reduce fatigue
	Combine upper- and lower-body exercises	Strengthen bones
		Increase endurance
Aerobic	Every-other-day routine	General health
	Short bouts several times a day	Increase energy
	Alternate brisk exercise with slow exercise to build up total duration of aerobic activity	Weight control
		Improve mood
		Sleep better
		Increase stamina
		Lower blood pressure
		Strengthen bone
		Relaxation

by building a routine of fifteen minutes of the flexibility exercises. When you can do fifteen minutes of continuous flexibility exercise, you will have the motion and endurance needed to include strengthening and aerobic exercise in your fitness program. Flexibility exercises are shown and described in Chapter 11.

Strengthening Exercises

Strengthening exercises, sometimes called resistance exercises, are important for everyone, especially for a person with arthritis. Joint swelling and pain can make muscles weak. Not using muscles because of stiffness and pain can also lead to weakness. Weak muscles are a special problem if you have arthritis because strong muscles help absorb shock, support joints, and protect you from injuries. Strong muscles also improve endurance, and the ability to safely walk, climb stairs, lift, and reach. Strengthening exercises are part of your fitness program and of good arthritis self-management.

Strengthening exercises ask your muscles to work a little harder than usual. When you ask your muscles to do a little more on a regular basis, your muscles gradually adapt to the extra work by getting stronger. Strengthening exercises add resistance (extra work) by using the weight of your body, extra weights you hold, or elastic bands. The secret of a good strengthening program is to "overload" your muscles just enough to get them to adapt, and not so much they are sore and stiff a day or two after you exercised.

If you have particular joint problems or have been told to protect certain joints, check with a therapist about what strengthening exercises are best and safest for you. If you have not been active in some time, it is best to build up to fifteen minutes of flexibility exercises before adding strengthening to your program. Strengthening exercises are shown and explained in Chapter 12.

Aerobic Exercises

Many people think that aerobic exercise is not for them. When they hear the word *aerobic,* they think of people in crazy clothes jumping around to loud music. It is important to understand that aerobic exercise does not mean just "aerobic dance." Aerobic exercise, also known as endurance or cardiovascular exercise, is any physical activity that uses the large muscles of your body in rhythmic, continuous motions. The most effective types of aerobic exercise use your whole body: walking, dancing, swimming, bicycling, mowing the lawn, or even raking leaves.

The purpose of aerobic exercise is to improve the ability of your heart, lungs, blood vessels, and muscles to work efficiently and effectively. You can do this by asking your body to do just a bit more aerobic exercise than it does now. Your body will adapt to a regular program of aerobic exercise by becoming more "aerobically fit."

When you are aerobically fit, your heart doesn't have to beat so fast and it can pump more blood out to your body with each beat. Your blood vessels can carry enough blood to deliver oxygen to all parts of your body, and your muscles can work longer and harder with less fatigue. You are at less risk for problems such as heart disease, high blood pressure, and diabetes. Aerobic exercise is the kind of exercise that helps control weight, improve sleep, strengthen bones, reduce depression and anxiety, and build endurance. Aerobic exercise is really quite a bargain when you think of all the benefits you can gain.

A fitness program needs to include some aerobic activities three to four days a week. Chapter 13 explains ways for you to include aerobic exercise in your fitness program, and gives guidelines for deciding how much to do and how hard to work.

How Much Exercise Is Enough?

How often you exercise, what you do, and how much you do depend on your health and fitness now and what you want to accomplish with exercise. When it comes to exercise, remember that more is not always better. It is important to know when you have reached your goal and can say, "This is right for me." Chapters 11, 12, and 13 will give you more information about exercise frequency, intensity, and duration. For now, you can see from the recommendations below that being able to exercise for better health or fitness is a real possibility for everyone.

How much exercise is enough for general health? To be active enough to be in the category of people who have less risk of heart disease, diabetes, and high blood pressure than people who are sedentary and do no physical activity, follow these guidelines:

EXERCISE RECOMMENDATION FOR HEALTH

Type of exercise: Aerobic exercise such as walking
Frequency: 3 to 5 days a week
Intensity: Low to moderate exertion
Duration: Total 20 to 30 minutes each exercise day (can be 5 minutes 4 times a day, or 10 minutes 3 times a day, if 30 minutes all at once is too much)

To increase your all-around fitness and see improvements in your flexibility, strength, endurance, and weight, you will need to gradually build your exercise program until you can follow these guidelines:

EXERCISE RECOMMENDATION FOR FITNESS

Types of Exercise: Flexibility, strengthening, aerobic

Frequency: Aerobic—3 to 4 days a week
Strengthening—2 to 3 days a week
Flexibility—3 to 7 days a week

Intensity: Aerobic—Moderate intensity
Strengthening—Low to moderate exertion

Duration: Aerobic—30 to 40 minutes
Strengthening—10 repetitions of 8 to 10 exercises

PREPARING TO EXERCISE

Figuring out how to make the commitment of time and energy to regular exercise is a challenge for everyone. If you have arthritis, you have even more challenges. You must take precautions and find a program that is safe and comfortable. You also have to understand how to adapt your exercise to changes in your arthritis and joint problems. Learning how much is enough before you've done too much is especially important.

Start by learning your arthritis needs. If possible, talk with your doctor and other professionals who understand your kind of arthritis. Get their ideas about special exercise needs and precautions. Read the section "Exercise Ideas for Specific Diseases" at the end of this chapter. Learn to be aware of your own body, and plan your activities accordingly. Your personal exercise program should be based on *your* current level of health and fitness, *your* goals and desires, *your* abilities and special needs, and *your* likes and dislikes. Deciding to improve your fitness, and feeling the satisfaction of success, has nothing to do with competition or comparing yourself to others.

Opportunities in Your Community

Most people who exercise regularly do so with at least one other person. Two or more people can keep each other motivated, and a whole class can build a feeling of camaraderie. On the other hand, exercising alone gives you the most freedom. You may feel that there are no classes that would work for you or no buddy to exercise with. If so, start your own program: As you progress, you may find that these feelings change.

The Arthritis Foundation and Arthritis Society sponsor exercise programs taught by trained instructors and developed specifically for people with arthritis. Consult your local chapter or branch office.

Most communities now offer a variety of exercise classes, including special programs for people over fifty, adaptive exercises, mall walking, fitness trails, and others. Check with the local Y, community and senior centers, parks and recreation programs, adult education, and community colleges. Many hospitals sponsor employee and community fitness and health promotion programs. There is a great deal of variation in the content of these programs, as well as in the professional experience of the exercise staff. By and large, the classes are inexpensive, and those in charge of planning are responsive to people's needs.

Health and fitness clubs usually offer aerobic studios, weight training, cardiovascular equipment, and sometimes a heated pool. For all these services they charge membership and class fees. Make sure you understand the financial commitment before you sign up. Ask about low-impact, beginners, and over-fifty exercise classes, both in the aerobic studio and in the pool. Gyms that emphasize weight lifting generally don't have the programs or personnel to help you with a flexible, all-around fitness program. These are some qualities you should look for:

▼ **Classes** that are designed for moderate- and low-intensity exercise. You should be able to observe classes and participate in at least one class before committing.

▼ **Instructors** who have qualifications and experience. Knowledgeable instructors are more likely to understand special needs and be willing and able to work with you.

▼ **Membership policies** that allow you to pay only for a session of classes, or let you "freeze" membership at times when you can't participate. Some fitness facilities offer different rates depending on how many services you use. Some use a "punch card" system which gives you lots of flexibility.

▼ **Facilities** that are easy to get to, park near, and enter. Dressing rooms and exercise sites should be accessible and safe, with professional staff on site.

▼ **A pool** that allows "free swim" times when the water isn't crowded. Also, find out the policy about children in the pool; small children playing and making noise may not be compatible with your needs.

▼ **Staff and other members** with whom you feel comfortable.

Putting Your Program Together

The best way to enjoy and stick with your exercise program is to suit yourself! Choose what you want to do, a place where you feel comfortable, and an exercise time that fits your schedule. A young mother with school-age children will find it difficult to stick with an exercise program that requires her to leave home for a five o'clock class. A retired man who enjoys lunch with friends and an afternoon nap is wise to choose an early- or midmorning exercise time.

Having fun and enjoying yourself are benefits of exercise that often go unmentioned. Too often we think of exercise as serious business. However, most people who stick with a program do so because they enjoy it. They think of their exercise as recreation rather than a chore. Start off with success in mind. Allow yourself time to get used to new experiences, and you'll probably find that you look forward to exercise.

Some well-meaning health professionals can make it hard for a person with arthritis to stick to an exercise program. You may have been prescribed exercises to do on your own at home (sometimes four times a day) for the rest of your life! What a lonely-sounding chore! No wonder so many people never start, or give up quickly. Not many of us make lifelong commitments to unknown projects. Experience, practice, and success are necessary to establish a habit. Follow the self-management steps in Chapter 7 to make beginning your program easier.

Making an exercise plan and keeping track of progress are important parts of a successful exercise program. After you have read Chapters 11–13, use the "Exercise Planner" on page 115 to develop and keep track of your program. If you want more room for your daily record, use something like the calendar on page 116 or keep an exercise journal.

Ensuring Your Program's Success

1. **Choose exercises you want to do.** Combine any activities your doctor or other professional recommends, with exercises from the next three chapters, and/or some of your favorites. Write them down.

2. **Talk to other people** with arthritis who are exercising. Discuss concerns and share successes. Solve your problems together.

3. **Choose the time and place to exercise.** Tell your family and friends your plan.

4. **Make a contract with yourself.** Decide how long you'll stick with these particular exercises. Six to twelve weeks is a reasonable time commitment for a new program.

5. **Make an Exercise Diary or calendar.** Leave space to write down your exercises, how long you do them, your heart rate, and your reactions. We've shown an example of a calendar on page 116. Put your diary where you can see it and fill it out every day.

6. **Do some self-tests.** You will find these at the end of the next three chapters. Record the date and results on the fitness planner.

7. **Start your program.** Remember to begin gradually if you haven't exercised in a while.

8. **Repeat the self-tests.** At the end of your time period, repeat the self-tests, record the results, and check the changes. Record your daily and weekly progress in your Exercise Diary. Repeat the self-tests every three to four weeks and record the results on your Exercise Planner.

9. **Revise your program. Look over your planner and diary for ideas.** Decide what you liked, what worked, and what made exercising difficult. Modify your program and contract for another few weeks. You may decide to change some exercises, the place or time you exercise, or your exercise partners.

10. **Reward yourself for a job well done.**

Keeping It Up

If you haven't exercised recently, you'll undoubtedly experience some new feelings and discomfort in the early days. It's normal to feel muscle tension and possibly tenderness around joints, and to be a little more tired in the evenings. Muscle or joint pain that lasts more than two hours after the exercise, or feeling tired into the next day, means that you probably did too much too fast. Don't stop; just exercise less vigorously or for a shorter time the next day.

When you do aerobic exercise, it's natural to feel your heart beat faster, your breathing speed up, and your body get warmer. Feeling short of breath, nauseated, or dizzy, however, is not what you want. If this happens to you, stop exercising and discontinue your program until you check with your doctor.

EXERCISE PLANNER

Dates: _____ to _____

The Plan

To exercise _____ *days a week for* _____ *minutes a day*

To do:

❑ **Flexibility/warm-up exercises**

❑ **Aerobic exercise** _____

❑ **Strengthening**

Goal

To improve:

❑ **Flexibility**   ❑ **Endurance**   ❑ **Strength**

❑ **Other** _____

Evaluation/Comments:

_____

_____

_____

EXERCISE RECORD

Week #	S	M	Tu	W	Th	F	S
1							
2							
3							
4							
5							
6							
7							
8							
9							
10							
11							
12							
13							
14							
15							

CALENDAR

Month: _____

Sunday	Monday	Tuesday	Wednesday	Thursday	Friday	Saturday

People who have arthritis have additional sensations to sort out. It can be difficult at first to figure out which come from arthritis and which come from exercise. Talking to someone else with arthritis who has had experience starting a new exercise program can be a big help. Once you've sorted out the new sensations, you'll be able to exercise with confidence.

Think of your head as the coach and your body as your team. For success, all parts of the team need attention. Be a good coach. Encourage and praise yourself. Design "plays" you feel your team can execute successfully. Choose places that are safe and hospitable. A good coach knows his or her team, sets good goals, and helps the team succeed. A good coach is loyal. A good coach does not belittle, nag, or make anyone feel guilty. Be a good coach to your team.

Besides a good coach, everyone needs an enthusiastic cheerleader or two. Of course, you can be your own cheerleader, but being both coach and cheerleader is a lot to do. Successful exercisers usually have at least one family member or close friend who actively supports their exercise habit. Your cheerleader can exercise with you, help you get other chores done, praise your accomplishments, or just consider your exercise time when making plans. Sometimes cheerleaders pop up by themselves, but don't be bashful about asking for a hand.

With exercise experience you develop a sense of control over yourself and your arthritis. You learn how to alternate your activities to fit your day-to-day needs. You know when to do less and when to do more. You know that a flare, or a period of inactivity in taking care of the arthritis, doesn't have to be devastating. You know how to get back on track again.

Give your exercise plan a chance to succeed. Set reasonable goals and enjoy your success. Stay motivated. When it comes to your personal fitness program, sticking with it and doing it your way makes you a definite winner.

EXERCISE IDEAS FOR SPECIFIC DISEASES

Everything we've suggested up to now applies to everyone with arthritis. Here are some additional exercise ideas and tips for people with specific diseases.

Osteoarthritis

Since osteoarthritis is primarily a problem with joint cartilage, an exercise program should include taking care of cartilage. Cartilage needs joint motion to stay healthy. In much the same way that a sponge soaks up and squeezes out water, joint cartilage soaks up nutrients and fluid, and gets rid of waste products by being squeezed when you move the joint. If the joint is not moved regularly, cartilage deteriorates. If the joint is continually compressed, as the hips and knees are by long periods of standing, the cartilage can't expand and soak up nutrients and fluid.

Any joint with osteoarthritis should be moved through its full range of motion several times daily to maintain flexibility and to take care of the cartilage. Judge your activity level so that pain is not increased. If hips and knees are involved, walking and standing should be limited to no more than two to four hours at a time, followed by at least an hour off your feet to give cartilage time to decompress. Good posture, strong muscles with good endurance, and shoes that absorb the shocks of walking are important ways to protect cartilage and reduce joint pain.

Rheumatoid Arthritis

People with rheumatoid arthritis should pay special attention to flexibility, strengthening, and appropriate use of their joints. Maintaining good posture and joint motion will help joints, ease pain, and avoid tightness. Arthritis pain and long periods spent sitting or lying down can quickly lead to poor posture and limited motion, even in the joints not affected by the arthritis. Be sure to include hand and wrist exercises in your daily program (see pages 128–130). A good time to do these is after washing dishes or during a bath when hands are warm and more limber.

Rheumatoid arthritis sometimes affects the bones in the neck. It is best to avoid extreme neck movements and not to put pressure on the back of the neck or head.

Stiffness in the morning can be a big problem. Flexibility exercises before getting up or during a hot bath or shower seem to help. A favorite way to get loosened up is to "stretch like a cat." Also, doing gentle flexibility exercises in the evening before bed can help reduce morning stiffness.

Ankylosing Spondylitis and Psoriatic Arthritis

Ankylosing spondylitis and psoriatic arthritis can result in loss of motion in the neck, back, and hips. Flexibility exercises, especially for the neck, spine, shoulders, and hips, as well as breathing and chest expansion, are important parts of the exercise program. Muscle strengthening exercises for back and hips are also needed to maintain erect posture. Correct head and neck posture is also extremely important to maintain good alignment and reduce pain with activity.

In these diseases, inflammation of muscles, tendons, and ligaments also occurs, making them vulnerable to injuries and sprains. Repeated inflammation can result in shortening and thickening of tissue around joints and lead to loss of motion. Therefore, it is extremely important to do regular flexibility exercises. Exercise gently, with slow controlled holding movements. Bouncing or jerking is dangerous.

The Achilles tendon or heel cord is especially at risk. Use the Achilles Stretch (page 137) to keep the heel cord and tissue covering the sole of the foot elastic. This helps reduce the chance of tendon tears, plantar fasciitis, heel pain, and heel spurs. Resting for some time each day on your stomach with your feet hanging over the end of the bed is another way to encourage good posture.

Stiffness in the neck and spine doesn't mean you can't be physically fit. Swimming is an excellent exercise. Swimming strengthens back, shoulders, and hips and provides a good cardiovascular workout. Use a snorkel and mask to allow you to swim without turning your head to breathe.

Systemic Lupus Erythematosus (SLE)

The fatigue and joint pains that so many people with SLE experience can be a major stumbling block to being active. These problems can be improved with a regular program of moderate exercise undertaken when the disease process is under control. A program that includes flexibility, strengthening, and aerobic exercise is appropriate. It is wise to avoid high-impact activities such as jumping or bouncing, especially if you're taking oral corticosteroids. If you start to have pain in your hip or groin, check with your doctor to make sure you are not having hip problems. Combining walking, bicycling, and swimming or pool exercise will give you a well-balanced program with maximum safety. Nighttime flexibility exercises may help reduce morning stiffness.

Raynaud's Phenomenon

If cold sensitivity or Raynaud's phenomenon is a problem, avoid extreme temperature changes when you plan your exercise. If you live where there are cold winters, develop a good interior exercise program. Some people have found that wearing disposable latex surgical gloves underneath a pair of regular gloves or mittens is useful. If you like water exercise but the water temperature is too cold for your hands, try putting on latex gloves before getting in the water.

Osteoporosis

Regular exercise at all ages plays an important part in preventing osteoporosis and in strengthening bones that already show signs of the disease. Endurance exercises such as walking are effective for strengthening bone. Strengthening exercises for back and stomach muscles are necessary for maintaining good posture and also help strengthen the spine.

You can help yourself with a regular exercise program that includes some walking and general flexibility and strengthening of your back and stomach muscles.

If you have osteoporosis or think that you may be at risk for this condition, here are some exercise precautions for you to remember:

▼ No heavy lifting.

▼ Avoid falls. Be careful on pool decks, waxed floors, icy sidewalks, or cluttered surfaces.

▼ Don't bend down to touch your toes when standing. This puts unnecessary pressure on your back. If you want to stretch your legs or back, lie on your back and bring your knees up toward your chest.

▼ Sit up straight, and don't slouch. Good sitting posture puts less pressure on the back.

▼ If your balance is poor or you feel clumsy, consider using a cane or walking stick when you're in a crowd or on unfamiliar ground.

Fibromyalgia

This condition can occur by itself or appear in people who also have other forms of arthritis. The symptoms are stiffness, fatigue, general aching, and extremely tender spots around the shoulders, upper back, hips, and knees. There are no signs of inflammation or joint involvement. Exercise for this condition is still being investigated. So far it seems that a general program that includes exercises to develop good posture, flexibility, and gentle strengthening and low to moderate aerobic exercise such as walking is the best approach. People with fibromyalgia often get worse after doing very vigorous exercise, but low- to moderate-intensity exercise can help reduce muscle tension, decrease pain, and aid relaxation.

REFERENCES

Ellert, Gwen. *Arthritis and Exercise: A User's Guide to Fitness and Independence.* Hignell Printing Ltd., 1988.

Francis, Peter, Ph.D., and Lorna Francis, Ph.D. *If It Hurts, Don't Do It.* Rocklin, Calif.: Prima Publishing and Communications, 1988. An easy-to-read book about getting started with an enjoyable and sensible fitness exercise program.

Lyons, Pat, R. N., and Debby Burgard. *Great Shape: The First Exercise Guide For Large Women.* New York: William Morrow/Arbor House, 1988.

Sayce, Valerie, and Ian Fraser. *Exercise Can Beat Your Arthritis.* In North America, from Avery Publishing Group: Garden City Park, NY, 1989. In Australia and New Zealand, from Fraser Publications, Melbourne, Victoria, 1987. Well-illustrated and explained exercises for the whole body.

▼ ▼ ▼ ▼ ▼ ▼ ▼

11. Flexibility Exercises

THIS chapter illustrates and explains flexibility exercises. Use these exercises to:

▼ Improve flexibility
▼ Get in shape for more vigorous exercise
▼ Keep the exercise habit on days when you don't do other kinds of exercise
▼ Warm up before and cool down after aerobic exercise

If you are not exercising regularly now, or if you have pain or stiffness that interferes with your daily activities, start your program with exercises from this chapter. Gradually build up the number and repetitions to a fifteen-minute session. When you can do a continuous fifteen minutes of flexibility exercises, gradually add strengthening and aerobic exercises (see Chapters 12 and 13). Choose exercises to build a program for the whole body.

Exercises are arranged in groups for different parts of the body. You can choose the positions and exercises that best suit you. Most of the upper-body exercises may be done either sitting or standing. Exercises done lying down can be performed on the floor or on a firm mattress. We've labeled the exercises that are particularly important for good posture "VIP" (very important for posture).

TIPS FOR FLEXIBILITY EXERCISES

Follow these helpful hints when you do flexibility exercises:

▼ Move slowly and gently. Do not bounce or jerk.
▼ To loosen tight muscles and limber up stiff joints, stretch just until you feel tension and then hold for a count of 15.
▼ Start with no more than five repetitions of any exercise. Take at least two weeks to increase to ten.

▼ Arrange your exercises so you don't have to get up and down a lot.

▼ Always do the same exercises for your left side as for your right.

▼ Breathe naturally. Do not hold your breath. Count out loud to make sure that you are breathing easily.

▼ If you have increased pain that lasts more than two hours after exercising, next time do fewer repetitions or eliminate an exercise that seems to be causing the pain. Don't stop exercising.

You might enjoy creating a routine of flexibility exercises that flow together and exercising to gentle, rhythmic music. Some people like to sprinkle flexibility exercises throughout the day to reduce stiffness and discomfort. Other people have found that doing a few flexibility exercises before bed reduces morning stiffness. If you are exercising to increase range of motion, remember to hold your position for about fifteen seconds at the point of feeling some tension.

NECK FLEXIBILITY EXERCISES

1. Chin In (VIP)

This exercise relieves jaw, neck and upper-back pain and is the start of good posture. You can do it while driving, sitting at a desk, sewing, reading, or exercising. Just sit or stand straight and gently slide your chin back. Keep looking forward as your chin moves backward. You'll feel the back of your neck lengthen and straighten. To help, put your finger on your nose and then draw straight back from your finger. (Don't worry about a little double chin—you really look much better with your neck straight!)

If it's uncomfortable for you to do this exercise at first, practice the movement lying flat on your back on the floor or on a firm mattress without a pillow. In this position, pull your chin in by pressing the base of your skull into the mattress. As your neck becomes more flexible, you will be able to hold this good head position comfortably when you are sitting and standing.

2. Two-Way Neck Stretch

In chin-in position (Exercise 1), and with your shoulders relaxed,

1. Turn slowly to look over your right shoulder. Then turn slowly to look over your left shoulder.
2. Tilt your head to the right and then to the left. Move your ear toward your shoulder. Do *not* move your shoulder up to your ear.

   If these exercises make you dizzy, close your eyes. If you are still dizzy, skip it. Don't do these exercises if they cause neck pain, or pain or numbness in your arms or hands.

SHOULDER AND ELBOW FLEXIBILITY EXERCISES

3. Shoulder Circles

You can do this exercise anytime to relax your shoulders and upper back. With shoulders relaxed and arms at your sides or hands resting in your lap, gently roll your shoulders forward, up, back, and down. Reverse and go the other way.

4. Sunrise Stretch (VIP)

You can do this stretch either sitting or standing.

1. Relax your arms, cross your wrists in front of you, and make gentle fists with your thumbs pointing down.
2. Start the movement with your hands. Roll your hands over, straighten fingers, move your arms upward and outward, and reach as high up as you can. Breathe in as you raise your arms.
3. Relax and return to the starting position, and breathe out as you bring your arms down.

This exercise encourages good posture and is a relaxing stretch for your upper body.

5. Bend and Reach

You can sit, stand, or lie on your back to do this exercise.

1. Start with your arms relaxed and elbows straight.
2. Bend your elbows to bring your hands up to touch your shoulders.
3. Then reach your hands up to the ceiling as you straighten your elbows. Reach as high as you can, stretching elbows and shoulders.
4. Breathe in as you stretch up and breathe out as you relax back to the starting position.

6. Pat and Reach

This double-duty exercise helps increase flexibility in both elbows and shoulders.

1. Raise one arm over your head and bend your elbow to pat yourself on the back.
2. Move your other arm to your back, bend your elbow, and reach up toward the other hand. Can your fingertips touch?
3. Relax and switch arm positions. Can you touch on that side? For most people, one position will work better than the other.

7. Shoulder Roll and Squeeze (VIP)

This is a good exercise to strengthen the middle and upper back and to stretch the chest.

1. Sit or stand with your head in chin-in position (Exercise 1) and your shoulders relaxed. Raise your arms out to the sides with elbows bent and fingertips pointed down.
2. Roll your hands upward until you are in a "stick 'em up" position.
3. Pinch your shoulder blades together by moving your elbows as far back as you can. Hold briefly. Relax.

If this exercise is uncomfortable, lower your arms below shoulder level.

8. Shoulder Pulley

Fasten a hook or pulley in a beam or on the top of a door frame. Place a piece of rope or clothesline through the hook, as shown. Start with enough rope to let you sit while exercising. Hold one end of the rope in each hand. If gripping the rope is uncomfortable, add padding or handles. As you pull down with one arm, the other arm will be raised. Move your arms up and down in front of you and also out to the side.

9. Wand Exercise

If one or both of your shoulders are particularly tight or weak, you may want to give yourself a "helping hand." This shoulder exercise and the next allow the arms to help each other.

Use a cane, yardstick, or mop handle as your wand. Place hands about shoulder width apart and raise the wand as high overhead as possible. You might try this in front of a mirror. This wand exercise can be done standing, sitting, or lying down.

HAND AND WRIST FLEXIBILITY EXERCISES

A good place to do these hand exercises is at a table that supports your forearms. Do them after washing dishes, after bathing, or as a break from handwork.

10. One-Two-Three Finger Exercises

For the best hand function, you should be able to make a loose fist with your thumb crossed over your fingers and to straighten your fingers completely. Use the one-two-three approach.

1. Begin bending the middle finger joints, then bend your knuckles so your fingertips are as close as possible to your palm.
2. Cross your thumb over your fingers toward your little finger.
3. Hold this position momentarily and then straighten your fingers and spread them wide apart. Use one hand to help the other if necessary.

11. Thumb Walk

Holding your wrist straight, form the letter O by lightly touching your thumb to each fingertip. After each O straighten and spread your fingers. Use the other hand to help if needed.

12. Hi and Bye (Hello and Cheerio)

1. To strengthen and limber your wrist, rest your forearm on a table with your hand over the edge. Keep fingers relaxed and bend your wrist up and down.
2. To strengthen the small muscles of the hand, slide your arm back until your fingers hang over with your knuckles at the table edge. Keeping your fingers straight and together and your palm flat, move your fingers up and down.

13. Door Opener

This is an exercise to stretch the muscles and ligaments that rotate the fore-arm, letting you turn doorknobs, use a screwdriver, or put your hand in your back pocket.

1. Start with your forearm resting on a table, palm down.
2. Keeping your upper arm and elbow tucked in close to your side and your little finger on the table, turn your hand so the palm faces up. Do not move your upper arm or elbow.

If you use your other hand to help, grip your forearm, not the wrist or hand.

TRUNK AND BACK FLEXIBILITY EXERCISES

14. Trunk Twist

You can do this stretch either sitting or standing. Move your arms to shoulder level or cross them over your chest. Slowly and gently twist at the waist to one side and then the other. Don't turn your head too far—this exercise is for your back. The purpose is to increase the flexibility of your trunk and make it easier and more comfortable for you to turn and roll. It will help loosen up your back to prepare for other exercise such as walking or dance.

15. Up and Over

This is a good stretch for trunk, shoulders, elbows, and hands. Sitting or standing, reach one arm up over your head and then reach with that hand over toward your other side, leaning your trunk slightly in that direction. You should feel a stretch along your trunk on the reaching side. Relax. Stretch your fingers out straight when you reach up and make a loose fist as you move back down. Do the same thing on the other side.

16. Pelvic Tilt (VIP)

This is an excellent exercise for your lower-back pain.

1. Lie on your back with your knees bent, feet flat. Place your hands on your abdomen.
2. Flatten the small of your back against the floor by tightening your stomach muscles and your buttocks. It helps to imagine bringing your pubic bone to your chin, or trying to pull your tummy in enough to zip a tight pair of trousers.
3. Hold the tilt for five to ten seconds. Relax.
4. Arch your back slightly. Relax.
5. Repeat the Pelvic Tilt. Keep breathing. Count the seconds out loud.

Once you've mastered the Pelvic Tilt lying down, practice it sitting, standing, and walking.

17. Lower-Back Rock and Roll

1. Lie on your back and pull your knees up to your chest with your hands behind the thighs. Rest in this position for ten seconds.
2. Gently roll knees from one side to the other, rocking your hips back and forth. Keep your upper back and shoulders flat on the ground.

18. Back Lift (VIP)

This exercise improves flexibility along your spine. Lie on your stomach and rise up onto your forearms. If this is comfortable, straighten your elbows. Breathe naturally and relax. If you have moderate to severe lower-back pain, do not do this exercise unless it has been specifically prescribed for you.

19. Knee-to-Chest Stretch

1. For a hip and lower-back stretch, lie on the floor with knees bent and feet flat.
2. Bring one knee toward your chest, using your hands to help.
3. Hold your knee near your chest for ten seconds and lower the leg slowly.
4. Repeat with the other knee.

To get more lower-back stretch, tuck both legs at the same time. Relax and enjoy the stretch.

20. Cat Back and Sway

This is a good way to loosen up your back and strengthen stomach muscles too.

1. On hands and knees, on forearms and knees, or leaning over a counter or table, relax and let your back sway and your stomach sag.
2. Slowly arch your back like a mad cat as you tighten and pull in your stomach.
3. Relax your back and let it sway again.
4. Repeat whole sequence.

Be sure to keep looking at the floor and to breathe naturally as you move back and forth from arch to sway.

HIP AND KNEE FLEXIBILITY EXERCISES

21. Hip Rolls

This is an important exercise to keep the hip flexible and in good positions for comfortable walking and standing up straight.

1. Stand with one foot slightly in front of the other. Slightly bend hip and knee of forward leg so that your heel is off the floor.
2. Keeping your foot in place and swiveling on your toes, roll your knee in then out. Although you can see your knee moving, the motion is really in your hip.

If you have hip pain when you stand on one foot, you can do this movement lying down (Hip Hooray, Exercise 23).

22. Back Kick (VIP)

This exercise increases the backward mobility and strength of your hip. Hold on to a counter for support. Move the leg up and back. Keep your knee fairly straight and do not point your toes. Stand tall and do not arch your back.

23. Hip Hooray

This exercise can be done lying on your back (A) or standing (B).

A. If you lie down, spread your legs as far apart as possible. Roll your legs and feet out like a duck and then in, pigeon-toed. Keep your knees straight.

B. If you are standing, move one leg out to your side as far as you can. Lead out and in with the heel. Hold on to a counter for support.

24. Hamstring Stretch

This exercise helps loosen tight hamstrings. Do the self-test for hamstring tightness (page 139) to see if you need to do this exercise. It is also a good exercise to do if you get muscle cramps in the back of your thigh. If you have unstable knees, or "back knee" (a knee that curves backward when you stand up), do not do this exercise.

A. 1. Lie on your back, knees bent, feet flat.
    2. Bend one hip so your leg is at about a right angle with the body.
    3. Slowly straighten the knee. Hold the leg as straight as you can as you count to 15.

B. You can also do this exercise by sitting with your foot on a low footstool. With your knee straight and toes pointed up, lean forward from the hips (back straight) until you feel a stretch on the back of your leg. Hold and count to 15. Relax.

Be careful with this exercise. It's easy to overstretch and be sore.

ANKLE AND FOOT FLEXIBILITY EXERCISES

Do these exercises sitting in a straight-backed chair with your feet bare. Have a bath towel and ten marbles or small paper wads next to you. These exercises are for flexibility, relaxation, and comfort.

25. Ankle Circles

With your heels on the ground, slowly circle your ankles to the right and then to the left. Go as far in each direction as you can.

26. Towel Grabber

1. Spread a towel out in front of your chair. Place your feet on the towel with your heels on the edge closest to you. Keep your heels down.
2. Scoot the towel back underneath your feet by pulling it with your toes as you arch your feet.
3. When you have done as much as you can, reverse the toe motion and scoot the towel out again.

You may do both feet together or separately.

27. Marble Pickup

Do this exercise one foot at a time. Place several marbles on the floor between your feet.

1. Keep your heel down and pivot your toes toward the marbles.
2. Pick up a marble in your toes and pivot your foot to drop the marble as far as possible from where you picked it up.
3. Repeat until all the marbles have been moved.
4. Reverse the process and return all the marbles to the starting position.

If marbles are difficult, try other objects like jacks, dice, or wads of paper.

28. Foot Roll

Place a rolling pin (or a large dowel or closet rod) under the arch of your foot and roll it back and forth. It feels great and stretches the ligaments in the arch of the foot.

29. Achilles Stretch

This exercise helps maintain flexibility in the Achilles tendon, and the large muscles you feel on the back of your calf. Good flexibility helps reduce the risk of injury, calf discomfort, and heel pain. The Achilles Stretch is especially helpful for cooling down after walking or cycling, and for people with ankylosing spondylitis or psoriatic arthritis. Also do this exercise if you get calf cramps.

1. Stand at a counter or against a wall. Place one foot in front of the other, toes pointing forward and heels on the ground.
2. Lean forward, bend the knee of the forward leg and keep the back knee straight, heel down. You will feel a good stretch in the calf.
3. Hold the stretch for 15 seconds. Do *not* bounce. Move gently.

It's easy to get sore doing this exercise. If you have worn shoes with high heels for a long time, be particularly careful.

THE WHOLE BODY

30. The Stretcher

This exercise is a whole-body stretch to do lying on your back. Start the motion at your ankles as explained here, or reverse the process if you want to start with your arms first.

1. Point your toes, and then pull your toes toward your nose. Relax.

2. Bend your knees. Then flatten your knees and let them relax.

3. Arch your back. Do the Pelvic Tilt (Exercise 16). Relax.

4. Breathe in and stretch your arms above your head. Breathe out and lower your arms. Relax.

5. Stretch your right arm above your head, and stretch your left leg by pushing away from you with your heel. Hold for a count of 10. Switch to the other side and repeat.

SELF-TESTS FOR FLEXIBILITY

Whatever our goals, we all need to see that our efforts make a difference. Since an exercise program produces gradual changes, it's often hard to tell if the program is working and to recognize improvement.

Choose several of these flexibility tests to measure your progress. Perform each test before you start your exercise program. Record the results. After every four weeks, do the tests again and check your improvement.

Make up some tests of your own, using motions or tasks that you would like to perform more easily, such as reaching a high shelf, tying a shoe, or scratching your back.

Test 1. Arm Flexibility

Do Exercise 6, Pat and Reach, for both sides of the body. Ask someone to measure the distance between your fingertips.

Goal: Less distance between your fingertips.

Test 2. Shoulder Flexibility

Stand facing a wall with your toes touching the wall. One arm at a time, reach up the wall in front of you. Hold a pencil, or have someone mark how far you reached. Also do this sideways, standing about three inches (8 cm) away from the wall.

    Goal: To reach higher.

Test 3. Hamstring Flexibility

Do the Hamstring Stretch, Exercise 24, one leg at a time. Keep your thigh perpendicular to your body. How much does your knee bend? How tight does the back of your leg feel?

    Goal: Straighter knee and less tension in the back of the leg.

Test 4. Ankle Flexibility

Sit in a chair with your bare feet flat on the floor and your knees bent at a 90-degree angle. Keep your heels on the floor. Raise your toes and the front of your foot. Ask someone to measure the distance between the ball of your foot and the floor.

    Goal: One to two inches (3 to 5 cm) between your foot and the floor.

▼ ▼ ▼ ▼ ▼ ▼ ▼

12. Strengthening Exercises

THE EXERCISES in this chapter make your muscles work against resistance and thus grow stronger. If you are not exercising regularly now, do not start with this chapter. Go to Chapter 11 and begin a program of flexibility exercises. Once you can do flexibility exercises for fifteen consecutive minutes, add strengthening exercises as well as aerobic activity (see Chapter 13). Choose exercises to build a program for the whole body. Always start your exercise session with some flexibility exercises to warm up; don't jump straight to strengthening or aerobic activity.

TIPS FOR STRENGTHENING EXERCISES

This chapter describes exercises for all parts of the body. The exercises for your trunk and legs use gravity, your body weight, or other muscles for resistance. The upper-body exercises use both hand-held weights and elastic bands as resistance; choose one of these methods, weights or bands. The exercises that are especially important for posture are labeled VIP.

Follow these tips as you plan your program of strengthening exercises:

▼ Start off doing no more than five repetitions.

▼ Gradually increase to no more than ten repetitions of eight to ten different exercises.

▼ Go slowly. Muscle soreness and stiffness often do not show up for twenty-four to forty-eight hours after the exercise.

▼ Always do the same exercises for your left side as for your right.

▼ Breathe naturally. Do not hold your breath. Count out loud to make yourself breathe.

▼ Two or three times a week is enough for strengthening exercises. Your muscles adapt and get stronger after the exercise, during the rest period, and before you do resistance exercise again. So it is important to give them time to improve.

BACK- AND ABDOMEN-STRENGTHENING EXERCISES

31. Back Up (VIP)

This exercise strengthens back muscles.

1. Lie on your stomach with your arms at your side or overhead.
2. Lift your head, shoulders, and arms. Do *not* look up. Keep looking down with your chin tucked in.
3. Count out loud as you hold for a count of 10. Relax.

    You can also lift your legs off the floor instead of your head and shoulders.

32. Curl-up (VIP)

A Curl-up, as shown here, will strengthen abdominal muscles. Lie on your back, knees bent, feet flat. Do the Pelvic Tilt (Exercise 16). Slowly curl up to raise your head and shoulders. Uncurl back down, or hold for ten seconds and slowly lower your shoulders and head. Keep your chin in.

Breathe out as you curl up, and breathe in as you go back down. Do *not* hold your breath. If you have neck problems, or if your neck hurts when you do this exercise, try the next one instead. Never tuck your feet under a chair or have someone hold your feet!

33. Roll-out

This is another good abdominal strengthener and easy on the neck. Use it instead of the Curl-up, or, if neck pain is not a problem, do them both. You strengthen your abdominal muscles by holding a Pelvic Tilt against the weight of your leg. Do not do this exercise if it causes hip or back pain.

1. Lie on your back with knees bent and feet flat. Bring one knee up to your chest.
2. Do the Pelvic Tilt (Exercise 16) and hold your lower back firmly against the floor.
3. Slowly and carefully, move one leg away from your chest as you straighten your knee. Move your leg out until you feel your lower back start to arch.
4. Tuck your knee back to your chest. Reset your pelvic tilt and roll your leg out again. Breathe out as your leg rolls out. Do *not* hold your breath.
5. Repeat with the other leg.

As you get stronger, you'll be able to straighten your legs out farther.

HIP STRENGTHENING EXERCISES

34. Back Kick (VIP)

This exercise increases the backward mobility and strength of your hip. Hold on to a counter for support. Move the leg up and back. Keep your knee fairly straight and do not point your toes. Stand tall and do not arch your back.

35. Leg Up

This is a good exercise to keep hips strong and in good position.

1. Lying on your stomach, raise one leg at a time up in the air. Bend the knee slightly if you wish, and keep the foot and ankle relaxed. Pointing your toes and bending your knee can lead to cramps.

2. Using your buttock muscles, raise your leg. Do not roll from side to side. Lower your leg slowly.

3. Raise the other leg. Your back may be more comfortable with a pillow under your stomach. If you are unable to lie on your stomach, you can do the movement standing (Back Kick, Exercise 34).

36. Ups and Downs

This is a good exercise to strengthen many muscles in your legs that are important for arising from a chair, climbing stairs, and walking.

1. Standing in front of a chair with arms at your sides or slightly in front of you, slowly bend hips and knees as if you were going to sit down.

2. Lower yourself only halfway, then straighten your hips and knees to stand back up again. Do not use your hands to help.

Do not lower yourself so far that you can't straighten back up by yourself or so far that your knees hurt. As you get stronger, you will be able to go farther down.

37. Side Kick

This exercise can be done either lying on your side (A) or standing (B). Do it lying down if standing on one leg makes your hip hurt.

A. Lying on your side, bend bottom leg and arm for support. Keep the upper leg straight and in line with your body. Raise the leg up in the air, keeping your knee and toes pointing straight forward. Hold briefly and relax. When you have finished one side, roll over to exercise the other side.

B. Stand using a chair or counter for support. Standing up straight and keeping your leg in line with your body, raise your leg out to the side, keeping knee and toes facing forward. Hold briefly and relax. Repeat on the other side.

KNEE- AND ANKLE-STRENGTHENING EXERCISES

38. Knee Strengthener (VIP)

Strong knees are important for walking, stair climbing, getting up and down, and standing comfortably. This exercise strengthens the knee. Sitting in a chair, straighten the knee by tightening up the muscle on top of your thigh. Place your hand on your thigh and feel the muscle work. Hold your knee as straight as possible. As your knee strengthens, see if you can build up to holding your leg out for thirty seconds. If straightening your knee from a fully bent position is uncomfortable, start with your foot resting on a low stool, as shown. Count out loud. Do *not* hold your breath.

39. Power Knees

This exercise strengthens the muscles that bend and straighten your knee.

1. Sit in a straight-backed chair and cross your legs above the ankles. Your legs can be almost straight, or you can bend your knees as much as you like. Try several positions.
2. Push forward with your back leg and press backward with your front leg. Exert pressure evenly so that your legs do not move.
3. Hold and count out loud for ten seconds. Relax.
4. Change leg positions. Be sure to keep breathing.

40. Ready-Set-Go

If you have painful knees, this is a good exercise to do when you first stand up.

1. Stand with one foot slightly in front of the other, heel of the forward leg on the ground, and toes off the ground (as if you are going to take a step).
2. Straighten and tighten the knee of the forward leg by tensing the muscles on the front of the thigh. Hold for a count of 5. Relax.
3. Say "Go" to yourself each time you tighten the muscles.

Try two or three "Go's" on each knee before you start to walk and then say "Go" to yourself each time your heel touches the floor to remind you to use your knee muscles correctly.

tighten this muscle

41. Tiptoes

This exercise will help strengthen your calf muscles and make walking, climbing stairs, and standing less tiring.

1. Hold on to a counter or table for support and rise up on your tiptoes. Hold for five seconds.
2. Lower slowly.

How high you go is not as important as keeping your balance and controlling your ankles. It is easier to do both legs at the same time. If your feet are too sore, wear shoes or do it while sitting down.

UPPER-BODY STRENGTHENING EXERCISES

Upper-Body Strengthening Exercises with Weights

Start with weights of no more than half a pound to 3 pounds (.25 to 1.5 kg). You should be able to complete at least eight repetitions with only mild fatigue. Exercise at a comfortable speed. Make sure that you relax after each motion. Count to make the periods of work and relaxation of equal length. Do strengthening exercises within your comfortable range of motion and remember to maintain good posture and normal breathing. Hand weights can be padded to increase the grip size. Some people like wrist weights because grasping is eliminated; however, these can be difficult to slip on over sore hands. Sometimes a home-made weight can solve problems best, for example, socks filled with sand or beans, or canned goods, or individual soda bottles.

42. Upright Row

1. Start with your arms relaxed in front of your body, with your hands together, and the palms facing the body.
2. Lift the hands straight up to chest level. The elbows bend and move out to the side and the hands stay together.

43. Lateral Lift

1. Start with your arms relaxed at your sides with the palms facing in.
2. Lift your arms up and out to the sides with elbows straight and palms facing down.

44. Triceps Press

Start with your elbow bent and your hand at your side at waist level. Bend slightly forward. Keep your upper arm steady and straighten your elbow.

45. Biceps Curl

Start with your arms relaxed at your sides and your palms facing forward. Keeping your upper arms steady, bend your elbows, bringing your hands up toward your shoulders.

Upper-Body Strengthening with Elastic Bands

Another way to strengthen muscles is to use large elastic bands for resistance. These are available from exercise classes, sports stores, and catalogues. The strength of the resistance varies, and you will want to try out the resistance that is best for you. Move through your comfortable range of motion and make sure you are in control. Do not let the band pull you around. Good posture and natural breathing are important when you do these exercises. A good goal is to gradually build up to repeating each exercise eight to ten times. Bands can be used as loops or with handles. Elastic bands can put a lot of stress on hands and wrists and may not be a good choice for everyone.

46. Horizontal Pull

1. Start with your arms out in front of you at shoulder level, with your elbows and wrists straight.

2. Keep your arms at shoulder level and move your hands apart, pulling your arms out to your sides. Relax.

47. Chest Press

1. Place the band across your back, resting it snugly over your shoulder blades. With your elbows bent, hold the ends of the band in front of each underarm. Your thumbs should be up, as when you hold a mug.
2. Straighten your elbows, pressing your arms forward. Relax.

48. Biceps Curl

1. Hold both ends of the band in one hand and put your foot through the loop that is formed, standing on the band.
2. Bend your elbow and bring your hand up toward your shoulder. Relax.
3. Repeat with the opposite arm.

SELF-TESTS

We all need to see that our efforts make a difference. Since an exercise program produces gradual change, it's often hard to tell whether the program is working and to recognize improvement. Choose several of these strength tests to measure your progress. Not everyone will be able to do all the tests. Choose those that work best for you. Perform each test before you start your exercise program. Record the results. After every four weeks, do the tests again and check your improvement.

Test 1. Grip Strength

Roll up a blood-pressure cuff and secure it with an elastic bandage or surgical tape. Have someone inflate the cuff to about 30 mm Hg and then squeeze as hard as you can in your fist. Record the readings for both hands.

> Goal: Stronger grip, higher readings.

Test 2. Abdominal Strength

Use the Curl-up, Exercise 32. Count how many repetitions you can do before you get too tired to do more, or count how many you can do in thirty seconds.

> Goal: More repetitions.

Test 3. Knee and Hip Strength

Count how many times in thirty seconds you can stand up from a chair and sit without using your hands.

> Goal: More repetitions, less fatigue.

Ask someone to time you and see how long it takes you to go up and down a flight of steps or walk 50 feet (15 meters).

> Goal: Less time, faster speed.

Test 4. Ankle Strength

This test has two parts. Stand at a table or counter for support.

Do Exercise 41, Tiptoes, as quickly and as often as you can. How many can you do in fifteen seconds?

Stand with your feet flat. Put most of your weight on one foot, and quickly tap the front part with your other foot. How many taps can you do in fifteen seconds?

Goal: More repetitions in each movement.

▼ ▼ ▼ ▼ ▼ ▼ ▼

13. Aerobic Activities

WHO NEEDS AEROBICS?

W E ALL need some aerobic exercise on a regular basis. If you walk, swim, do aquaerobics, bicycle, or walk when you golf, you are doing aerobic exercise. Aerobic exercise is any physical activity that requires you to continuously move your arms and/or legs for at least five minutes. Regular aerobic exercise helps protect us from heart disease, high blood pressure, and diabetes. Aerobic exercise also helps us to control our weight, sleep well, and feel relaxed, energetic and happy. This chapter contains suggestions for different kinds of aerobic exercise and ideas for putting together an aerobic exercise program of your own.

YOUR AEROBIC EXERCISE PLAN

One of the biggest problems with aerobic exercise is that you may overdo it. Inexperienced exercisers think they have to work very hard for exercise to do any good. Exhaustion, sore muscles, and painful joints are the result of jumping in too hard and too fast. Finding the aerobic exercise plan that is right for you doesn't need to be a guessing game. Use the following guidelines as you plan your aerobic exercise.

The Warm-up

Always warm up before your aerobic exercise. A warm-up raises the temperature in your muscles and joints, increases flexibility, increases circulation, and safely prepares your heart to work harder. A warm-up routine consists of flexibility exercises and a gradual increase in your aerobic activity level. Flexibility exercises prepare your muscles and joints for more vigorous activity and ready your heart and lungs for more work.

A good warm-up routine can consist of ten or fifteen minutes of flexibility exercises and five minutes of easy all-body movements. Examples of the all-body warm-ups are slow walking before a more vigorous aerobic walk, slow dancing before moving to faster music, or pedaling the bicycle at a slower speed and with no resistance before you go on to a more energetic ride.

The Cool-down

A short five- to ten-minute cool-down period after you have finished a more vigorous activity is important to help your body gradually return to a resting state. The cool-down gives your heart a chance to slow down gradually; your body, to lose some of the heat you generated during exercise; and your muscles, to relax and stretch out.

To cool down, continue your aerobic exercise in slow motion for three to five minutes. For example, after a brisk walk, cool down with a casual stroll. End a bicycle ride with slow easy pedaling. The cool-down is a good time to do some flexibility exercises because your muscles and joints are warm and less stiff. Gentle flexibility exercises during cool-down help reduce muscle soreness that sometimes follows vigorous activity. If you have been walking or bicycling be sure to include the Achilles Stretch (Exercise 29, page 137).

Frequency: How Often?

Three or four times a week is the best frequency for aerobic exercise. Taking every other day off gives your body a chance to rest and adapt.

Duration: How Long?

If you have not been active in a while, start your aerobic exercise with no more than five minutes at a time. You can exercise five minutes several times a day and gradually increase the duration of your aerobic activity to about thirty minutes a session, or continue to spread it out over the day. You can also safely increase the duration of your aerobic exercise by alternating periods of brisk and easy exercise. For example, walk slowly for three to five minutes, then walk briskly for the same amount of time, and then slow down again. Eventually you can build up to longer periods of brisk exercise and use the slow periods as warm-ups and cool-downs.

Intensity: How Hard?

Safe and effective aerobic exercise should be done at no more than moderate intensity. High-intensity exercise increases the risk of injury and causes discomfort, so not many people stick with it. Exercise intensity is measured by how hard you work. For a trained runner, completing a mile in ten minutes is probably low-intensity exercise. For a person who hasn't exercised in a long time, a brisk ten-minute walk may be moderate to high intensity. The trick, of course, is to figure out what is moderate intensity for you. There are several easy ways to do this.

Perceived Exertion: An easy and reliable way to monitor intensity is to rate how hard you feel you're working on a scale of 0 to 10. Zero, at the low end of the scale, is lying down, doing no work at all. Ten is equivalent to working as hard as possible—very hard work that you couldn't do longer than a few seconds. Of course, you never want to exercise that hard. A good level for aerobic exercise is between 3 and 5 on this scale.

PERCEIVED EXERTION SCALE
How Does the Exercise Feel?

NUMBERS	RATING
0	Nothing at all
1	Very Weak
2	Weak
3	Moderate
4	Somewhat Strong
5	Strong
6	
7	Very Strong
8	
9	
10	Very, Very Strong

Heart Rate: Unless you're taking heart-regulating medication, monitoring your pulse while exercising is a good way to measure exercise intensity. The faster the heart beats, the harder you're working. (Your heart also beats fast when you are frightened or nervous, but here we're talking about how your heart responds to physical activity.) Aerobic exercise at moderate intensity raises your heart rate into a range between 60% and 80% of your maximum heart rate. Maximum heart rate declines with age, so your safe exercise heart rate gets lower as you get older. You can use the Suggested Exercise Heart Rate chart to find your exercise heart rate.

If you want to use heart rate to guide your exercise, you need to know how to take your pulse. You'll need a clock with a second hand. Take your pulse by placing the pads of your middle three fingers at your wrist below the base of your thumb. Don't use the tips of your fingers, and don't use your thumb. You should be able to feel your blood pumping. Count how many beats you feel in fifteen seconds. Multiply this number by 4 to find out how fast your heart is beating in one minute. Start taking your pulse whenever you think of it, and you'll soon learn the difference between your resting and exercise heart rates.

SUGGESTED EXERCISE HEART RATE, BY AGE

AGE RANGE	PULSE (NUMBER OF HEARTBEATS IN 15 SECONDS)
20–30	30–38
30–40	28–36
40–50	26–34
50–60	24–32
60–70	22–30
70–80	20–28
80 +	18–24

The most important reason for knowing your exercise heart rate range is so that you can learn not to exercise too vigorously. After you've done your warm-up and five minutes of aerobic activity, take your pulse. If it's higher than the upper rate on the chart, slow down. Don't work so hard. If you are a beginning exerciser, keep your exercise heart rate down at the lower end of the range shown on the Suggested Exercise Heart Rate chart.

At first some people have trouble getting their heart rate up to the lower rate. Don't worry about that. Keep exercising at a comfortable level. As you get more experienced and stronger your heart rate will rise, because you can exercise more vigorously.

If you are taking medicine that regulates your heart rate, have trouble feeling your pulse, or think that keeping track of your heart rate is a bother, use one of the other methods to monitor your exercise intensity.

Talk Test: Talk to another person or yourself, sing, or recite poems while you exercise. Moderate-intensity exercise allows you to speak comfortably. If you can't carry on a conversation or sing to yourself because you are breathing too hard or are short of breath, you're working too hard. Slow down. The talk test is an easy way to regulate exercise intensity.

Remember to follow the guidelines on frequency, duration, and intensity. Sometimes you need to tell yourself (and maybe others) that enough is enough. More exercise is not necessarily better, especially if it gives you pain or discomfort. As *The Walking Magazine* said, "Go for the smiles, not the miles."

WALKING

You can walk to condition your heart and lungs, strengthen bones and muscles, relieve tension, control weight, and generally feel good. Walking is easy, inexpensive, safe, and accessible. You can walk by yourself or with company, and you can take your exercise with you wherever you go. Walking is safer and puts less stress on the body than jogging or running. It's an especially good choice if you are older, have been sedentary, or have joint problems.

Most people with arthritis can walk as a fitness exercise. If you walk to shop, visit friends, and do household chores, then you'll probably be able to walk for exercise. Using a cane or walker need not stop you from getting into a walking routine. If you are in a wheelchair, use crutches, or experience more than mild discomfort when you walk a short distance, you should consider some other type of aerobic exercise, or consult a physician or therapist for help.

Be cautious during the first two weeks of walking. If you haven't been doing much for a while, ten minutes of walking may be enough. Build up your time with intervals of strolling. Each week increase the brisk walking interval by no more than five minutes until you are up to twenty or thirty minutes. Follow the frequency, duration, and intensity guidelines, and read these tips on walking before you start.

Walking Tips

1. **Choose your ground.** Walk on a flat, level surface. Walking on hills, uneven ground, soft earth, sand, or gravel is hard work and often leads to hip, knee, or foot pain. Fitness trails, shopping malls, school tracks, streets with sidewalks, and quiet neighborhoods are good places to get started.

2. **Always warm up and cool down with a stroll.** It's important to walk slowly for three to five minutes to prepare your circulation and muscles for a brisk walk, and to finish up with the same slow walk to let your body slow down gradually. Experienced walkers know they can avoid shin and foot discomfort when they begin and end with a stroll.

3. **Set your own pace.** It takes practice to find the right walking speed. To find your speed, start walking slowly for a few minutes, then increase your speed to a pace that is slightly faster than normal for you. After five minutes take your pulse and see if you are within your exercise heart rate range. If you are above the range or feel out of breath, slow down. If you are below the range, try walking a little faster. Walk another five minutes and take your pulse again. If you are still below your exercise range, don't try to raise your heart rate by walking uncomfortably fast. Keep walking at a comfortable speed and take your pulse in the middle and at the end of each walk.

4. **Increase your arm work.** You can also raise your heart rate into exercise range by bending your elbows a bit and swinging your arms more vigorously. Alternatively, carry a one- or two-pound (.5 to 1 kg) weight in each hand. You can purchase hand weights for walking, hold a can of food in each hand, or put sand, dried beans, or pennies in two small plastic beverage bottles or socks. The extra work you do with your arms increases your heart rate without forcing you to walk faster than you find comfortable.

Shoes

It's not necessary to spend a lot of money on shoes. Wear shoes of the correct length and width with shock-absorbing soles and insoles. Make sure they're big enough in the toe area: The "rule of thumb" is a thumb width between the end of your longest toe and the end of the shoe. You shouldn't feel pressure on the sides or tops of your toes. The shoe should hold your heel firmly when you walk so your heel doesn't slip up and down.

Wear shoes with a continuous crepe or composite sole in good repair. Shoes with leather soles and a separate heel don't absorb shock as well as the newer athletic and casual shoes. Shoes with laces or Velcro let you adjust width as needed and give more support than slip-ons. If you have problems tying laces, consider Velcro closures or elastic shoelaces.

Many people like shoes with removable insoles that can be exchanged for ones that are more shock absorbing. Insoles are available in sporting-goods stores and shoe stores. When you shop for insoles, take your walking shoes with you. Try on the shoe with the insole to make sure that there's still enough room inside for your foot to be comfortable. Insoles come in sizes and can be trimmed with scissors for a final fit. If your toes take up extra room, try the three-quarter insoles that stop just short of your toes. If you have prescribed inserts in your shoes already, ask your doctor or orthotist about insoles.

Possible Problems

1. If you have pain around your shins when you walk, you may not be spending enough time warming up. Do the ankle flexibility and strengthening exercises (pages 136-137) before you start walking (pages 145-147). Start your walk at a slow pace for at least five minutes. Keep your feet and toes relaxed.

2. Another common problem is sore knees. Fast walking puts more stress on knee joints. To slow your speed and keep your heart rate up, try doing more work with your arms (see above). Do the knee strengthening exercises (Exercises 38 and 39 on page 145) in your warm-up to help reduce knee pain.

3. Cramps in the calf and heel pain can often be eliminated by doing the Achilles Stretch (Exercise 29 on page 137) before and after walking. A slow walk to warm up also is helpful. If you have circulatory problems in your legs and experience cramps while walking, alternate intervals of brisk and slow walking. If this doesn't help, check with your physician or therapist for suggestions. Dehydration can also cause leg cramps. Make sure you increase your fluid intake while exercising.

4. Maintain good posture. Use the Chin In position (Exercise 1) and keep your shoulders relaxed to help reduce neck and upper back discomfort.

SWIMMING

Swimming is another good aerobic exercise. The buoyancy of the water lets you move your joints through their full range of motion and strengthen your muscles and cardiovascular system with less joint stress than on land. Swimming uses the whole body. If you haven't been swimming for a while, consider a refresher course.

To make swimming an aerobic exercise, you will eventually need to swim continuously for twenty minutes. Use the frequency, duration, and intensity guidelines to build up your endurance. Try different strokes, modifying them or changing strokes after each lap or two. This lets you exercise all joints and muscles without overtiring any one area.

Swimming Tips

1. **Use a mask and snorkel for breathing.** The breast stroke and crawl require a lot of neck motion and may be uncomfortable if you have neck pain. To solve this problem, use a mask and snorkel to breathe without twisting your neck.
2. **Swim goggles protect eyes.** Chlorine can be irritating to eyes. A good pair of goggles will protect your eyes and let you keep your eyes open while you're swimming.
3. **Take a hot shower or soak in a hot tub after your workout.** The warmth helps reduce stiffness and muscle soreness that may come from being in cool water.
4. **Always swim where there are qualified lifeguards.**

If you don't like to swim or are uncomfortable learning strokes, you can walk laps in the pool, or join the millions who are aquacizing.

AQUACIZE

Exercising in the water is comfortable, fun, and effective as a flexibility, strengthening, and aerobic activity. The buoyancy of the water takes weight off hips, knees, feet, and back. People who have trouble walking for endurance can usually aquacize. The pool is a good place to do your own routine, because no one can see you much below shoulder level.

Getting Started

Joining a water exercise class with a good instructor is an excellent way to get started. The Arthritis Foundation and Arthritis Society sponsor water exercise classes and train instructors. Contact your local chapter or branch office to see what is available. Many communities and private health clubs offer water exercise classes, with some geared to older adults.

If you have access to a pool and want to exercise on your own, there are many water exercise books available. One we recommend is *Hydrorobics,* which contains a lot of good ideas for exercise in the water (listed under "References" at the end of this chapter).

Water temperature is always a topic when people talk about water exercise. The U.S. Arthritis Foundation recommends a pool temperature of 84°F (29°C) with the surrounding air temperature in the same range. Except in warm climates, this means a heated pool. If you're just starting to aquacize, find a pool with these temperatures. If you can exercise more vigorously and don't have Raynaud's phenomenon or other cold sensitivity, you can probably aquacize in cooler water. Many pools where people swim laps are about 80°F to 83°F (27°C to 28°C). It feels quite cool when you first get in, but starting off with water walking, jogging, or another whole-body exercise helps you warm up quickly.

The deeper the water you stand in, the less stress there is on joints; however, a water level above midchest can make it hard to keep your balance. You can let the water cover more of your body just by spreading your legs apart or bending your knees a bit.

Aquacize Tips

1. **Protect your feet.** Wear something on your feet to protect them from rough pool floors and to provide traction in the pool and on the deck. Choices vary from terry cloth slippers with rubber soles (they stretch in water, so buy a size smaller than your shoe size) to footgear especially designed for water exercise. Some styles have Velcro tape to make them easier to put on. Beach shoes with rubber soles and mesh tops also work well. Do not wear thong sandals around or in a pool.

2. **Keep warm.** If you are sensitive to cold or have Raynaud's phenomenon, wear a pair of disposable latex surgical gloves. Boxes of gloves are available at most pharmacies. The water trapped and warmed inside the glove seems to insulate the hand. If your body gets cold in the water, wear a T-shirt and/or full-leg Lycra exercise tights for warmth.

3. **Try a step stool for easier access.** If the pool does not have steps, and it is difficult for you to climb up and down a ladder, try positioning a three-step kitchen stool in the pool by the ladder rails. This is an inexpensive way to provide steps for easier entry and exit, and it is easy to remove and store when not needed.

4. **Add more buoyancy.** Wearing a flotation belt or life vest adds extra buoyancy, to take weight off hips, knees, and feet. That makes exercising more comfortable for these joints.

5. **Regulate exercise intensity.** You can regulate how hard you work in the water by how you move. To make the work easier, move more slowly. Another way to regulate exercise intensity is to change how much water you push when you move. For example, when you move your arms back and forth in front of you under water, it is hard work if you hold your palms facing each other and clap. It is easier if you turn your palms down and slice your arms back and forth with only the narrow edge of your hands pushing against the water.

BICYCLING

Outdoor Bicycling

Cyclists who travel outdoors can enjoy the scenery and get out into the fresh air and sunshine. But they also face the risks of streets and bike paths, especially the danger of falling. Falls from bicycles can be serious. If you have problems with balance, vision, or hearing, or if you have osteoporosis, outdoor bicycling may not be for you. Consider a stationary bicycle instead (see the next section).

If you live in a flat area, consider an adult tricycle. Though heavy and harder to pedal than a bicycle, tricycles are very stable. The large basket makes it easy to run errands and carry packages.

Finding the Right Bicycle: A bicycle that is the proper size for you, and that is properly adjusted is essential. Incorrect seat height is the most common problem. It is also the easiest adjustment to make. To check seat height, have someone hold the bike while you sit on the seat. With your *heel* on the pedal, straighten your leg to the bottom of the pedal stroke. If your knee is still bent, the seat is too low. Keeping your knees bent while pedaling can cause knee pain. (People whose knees bend backward should leave just a little bend.) If you can't keep your heel on the pedal when the pedal is at its lowest point, you need to lower the seat.

Try different kinds of handlebars, gears, and brakes to find the styles that suit you best. Many bicycle shops can customize a bike to combine the features you want. Reading, talking to other bicyclists, and taking a trip to a bike shop will help you decide on your kind of bike. Once you know the features you

want, you may be able to find what you want at a yard sale or through a classified ad. Just get a professional safety check and tune-up before you ride.

Whatever style you choose, remember that bicycling uses different muscles
than walking. Don't be surprised if a five- or ten-minute ride is enough at first.
Follow the guidelines of frequency, duration, and intensity to progress gradually to twenty or thirty minutes of safe and enjoyable bicycling.

Riding Tips

1. **Wear a helmet.** The most important piece of equipment for bicycle riding
   is a helmet. Any fall can cause serious head injury. Don't risk it. There are
   ventilated helmets that weigh less than eight ounces (224 g). Look for a
   sticker showing that the helmet has been approved by a safety board,
   such as SNELL or ANSI in the United States.
2. **Follow the rules.** Learn and obey the bicycle road rules for your community. Take advantage of roads with a designated bicycle lane.
3. **Pedal with the *ball* of your foot.**
4. **Use gears correctly for safety and comfort.** Learn to use your gears so that
   you don't grind them. If you work hard to pedal and start to feel pain
   around your kneecap, you probably need to shift to a lower gear.

Stationary Bicycles

Stationary bicycles offer the fitness benefits of outdoor bicycling without the
outdoor hazards. They're preferable for people who don't have the flexibility
or strength to be comfortable pedaling and steering on the road. If you live in
a cold or hilly area, you may want to avoid the extra exertion of cycling
outdoors. Stationary bicycling is good to alternate when combined with other
kinds of aerobic exercise to provide choices between indoor and outdoor,
solitary and group, and weight-bearing and non-weight-bearing exercise.

Choosing a Bicycle: A wide variety of stationary bicycles is available. Most
models have a speedometer and odometer to show the speed and distance. Some
take your pulse by means of an ear clip or finger rings and give a digital readout.
Models at health clubs may have computer programs and video displays to take
you over hills and dales. There are also recumbent bicycles that place hips and
knees at about the same height. Some people find these the most comfortable.

The most important features that differ from model to model are:

1. **Seat.** Both regular bicycle and bench-style seats are available. Seats can be
   adjusted vertically or both vertically and horizontally. Adjust the seat so

that your knee is straight when your *heel* is on the pedal at the pedal's lowest point. If your knees are unstable or loose, or bend backward, adjust the seat height so that there is a little bend left in your knee, rather than having your legs be completely straight. If your knees don't straighten all the way, adjust the seat so that they are comfortably straight.

2. **Handlebars.** Stationary handlebars are for balance and for supporting your arms. Movable handlebars let you exercise the upper body. Using your arms as you exercise helps you spread the work out, instead of depending on your legs to do it all. You should be able to grip the handlebars without reaching or stretching, and with a slight bend in your elbows.

3. **Resistance.** How hard you have to push to turn the pedals can be adjusted with a dial or screw. On some models a fan wheel increases resistance as you pedal faster. If the resistance adjustment is manual, make sure you can easily reach and turn the control.

A loan or rental is a good way to start using a stationary bicycle. The classified ads are a great place to shop for your own. Not all models fit everyone, so try out any bicycle you are considering. Make sure it adjusts to positions that are comfortable and safe for you. Check all the points below.

▼ The bicycle is steady when you get on and off.
▼ The resistance is easy to set, and can be set to zero.
▼ The seat is comfortable.
▼ The seat can be adjusted for full knee extension when the pedal is at its lowest point.
▼ Large pedals and loose pedal straps allow feet to shift easily while you are pedaling.
▼ There is ample clearance from the frame for knees and ankles.
▼ The handlebars allow good posture and comfortable arm position.

Make It Interesting: The most common complaint about riding a stationary bike is that it's boring. If you ride while watching television, reading, or listening to music, you can become fit without being bored. One woman keeps interested by mapping out tours of places she would like to visit and then charts her progress on the map as she rolls off the miles. Other people set their bicycle time for the half hour of soap opera or news that they watch every day. There are videocassettes of exotic bike tours that put you in the rider's perspective. Book racks that clip on to the handlebars make reading easy.

Riding Tips

1. **Don't use too much resistance.** Bicycling uses different muscles from walking. Until your leg muscles get used to pedaling, you may only be able to ride a few minutes. Start off with no resistance. If you wish, increase resistance slightly every two weeks. Increasing resistance has the same effect as bicycling up hills. If you use too much resistance, your knees are likely to hurt, and you'll have to stop before you get the benefit of an aerobic exercise.

2. **Pedal at a comfortable speed.** For most people, fifty to sixty revolutions per minute (rpm) is a good place to start. Some bicycles tell you the rpm, or you can count the number of times your right foot reaches its lowest point in a minute. As you get used to bicycling, you can increase your speed. However, faster is not necessarily better. Listening to music at the right tempo makes it easier to pedal at a consistent speed. Experience will tell you the best combination of speed and resistance.

3. **Progress gradually at moderate intensity.** Set your goal for twenty to thirty minutes of pedaling at a comfortable speed. Build up your time by alternating intervals of brisk pedaling with less exertion. Use your heart rate, perceived exertion, or the talk test to make sure you aren't working too hard. If you're alone, try singing songs as you pedal. If you get out of breath, slow down.

4. **Chart progress.** Keep a record of the times and distances of your "bike trips." You'll be amazed at how much you can do.

5. **Keep the exercise habit.** On bad days, or if you have a painful knee, keep your exercise habit going by pedaling with no resistance, at fewer rpm, or for a shorter period of time.

The stationary bicycle is a particularly good alternative exercise. It does not put weight on your hips, knees, and feet, you can easily adjust how hard you work, and weather doesn't matter. Use the bicycle on days when you don't want to walk or do more vigorous exercise, or can't exercise outside.

OTHER EXERCISE EQUIPMENT

If you have trouble getting on or off a stationary bicycle, or don't have room for a bicycle where you live, you might try a restorator or arm crank. To purchase one, ask your therapist or doctor, or call a medical equipment supplier.

A restorator is a small piece of equipment with foot pedals that can be attached to the foot of a bed or a chair. It allows you to exercise by pedaling. Resistance can be varied, and placement of the restorator lets you adjust for leg length and knee bend. The restorator can be the first step in getting an exercise program started.

Arm cranks are bicycles for the arms. They are mounted on a table. People who are unable to use their legs for active exercise can improve their cardiovascular fitness by using the arm crank. It's important to work closely with a therapist to set up your program, because using only your arms for aerobic exercise requires different intensity monitoring from using the bigger leg muscles.

There is a wide variety of exercise equipment in addition to what we've mentioned so far. These include treadmills (self-powered and motor-driven), rowing machines, cross-country skiing machines, minitrampolines, and stair-climbing machines. Most are available in both commercial and home models. If you're thinking about exercise equipment, have your objectives clearly in mind. For cardiovascular fitness and endurance, you want equipment that will help you exercise as much of your body at one time as possible. The motion should be rhythmical, repetitive, and continuous. The equipment should be comfortable, safe, and not stressful on joints. If you're interested in a new piece of equipment, try it out for a week or two before buying it.

Exercise equipment that requires you to use weights usually does not improve cardiovascular fitness. A weight-lifting program builds strength, but it can put excessive stress on joints, muscles, tendons, and ligaments if done incorrectly. It is extremely important that you confer with your doctor or therapist when planning any program that uses weights or weight machines.

LOW-IMPACT AEROBIC DANCE

Most people find low-impact aerobic dance a safe and acceptable form of exercise. "Low-impact" means that one foot is always on the floor and there is no jumping. However, low-impact does not necessarily mean low-intensity, nor do the low-impact routines protect all joints. If you participate in a low-impact aerobic dance class, you'll probably need to make some modifications for your arthritis.

Getting Started

Start off by letting the instructor know who you are, that you may modify some movements to meet your needs, and that you may need to ask for advice. It's easier to start off with a newly formed class than it is to join an ongoing class. If you don't know people, try to get acquainted. Be open about why you may sometimes do things a little differently. You'll be more comfortable and may find others who also have special needs.

Most instructors use music or count to a specific beat, and do a set number of repetitions. You may find that the movement is too fast or that you don't want to do as many repetitions. Modify the routine by slowing down to half-time, or keep up with the beat until you start to tire and then slow down. If the class is doing an exercise that involves arms and legs and you get tired, try resting your arms and only doing the leg movements, or just walk in place until you are ready to go again. Most instructors will be able to instruct you in "chair aerobics" if you need some time off your feet.

Many low-impact routines use lots of arm movements done at or above shoulder level to raise heart rates. For people who have shoulder problems or high blood pressure, too much arm exercise above shoulder level can cause problems. Modify the exercise by lowering your arms or giving your arms frequent rests.

Being different from the group in a room walled with mirrors takes courage, conviction, and a sense of humor. The most important thing you can do for yourself is to choose an instructor who encourages everyone to exercise at his or her own pace and a class where people are friendly and having fun. Observe classes, speak with instructors, and participate in at least one class session before making any financial commitment.

Aerobic Studio Tips

1. **Wear supportive shoes.** Many studios have cushioned floors and soft carpeting that might tempt you to go barefoot. Don't! Shoes help protect the small joints and muscles in your feet and ankles by providing a firm, flat surface on which to stand.

2. **Protect your knees.** Stand with knees straight but relaxed. Many low-impact routines are done with bent, tensed knees and a lot of bobbing up and down. This can be painful and is unnecessarily stressful to your knees. Avoid this by remembering to keep your knees relaxed (aerobics instructors call this "soft" knees). Watch in the mirror to see that you keep the top of your head steady as you exercise. Don't bob up and down.

3. **Don't overstretch.** The beginning (warm-up) and end (cool-down) of the session will have stretching and strengthening exercises. Remember to stretch only as far as you comfortably can. Hold the position and don't

bounce. If the stretch hurts, don't do it. Ask your instructor for a less stressful substitute, or choose one of your own.

4. **Change movements.** Do this often enough so that you don't get sore muscles or joints. It's normal to feel some new sensations in your muscles and around your joints when you start a new exercise program. However, if you feel discomfort doing the same movement for some time, change movements or stop for a while and rest.

5. **Alternate kinds of exercise.** Many exercise facilities have a variety of exercise opportunities: equipment rooms with cardiovascular machines, pools, and aerobic studios. If you have trouble with an hour-long aerobic class, see if you can join the class for the warm-up and cool-down and use a stationary bicycle or treadmill for your aerobic portion. Many people have found that this routine gives them the benefits of both an individualized program and group exercise.

SELF-TESTS FOR AEROBIC FITNESS

It's important to see that your exercise program is making a measurable difference. Choose one of these aerobic fitness tests to perform before you start your exercise program. Pick the test that works best for you. Record your results. After four weeks of exercise, do the test again and check your improvement. Measure yourself after four more weeks. For ideas on other self-tests, see the book *If It Hurts, Don't Do It*, listed under "References" at the end of this chapter.

Test 1. Distance Test

Find a place to walk or bicycle where you can measure distance. A running track works well. On a street you can measure distance with a car. A stationary bicycle with an odometer provides the equivalent measurement. If you plan on swimming, you can count lengths of the pool.

After a warm-up, note your starting point and either bicycle, swim, or walk as briskly as you comfortably can for five minutes. Try to move at a steady pace for the full time. At the end of five minutes, mark your spot and immediately take your pulse and rate your perceived exertion from 0 to 10. Continue at a slow pace for three to five more minutes to cool down. Measure and record the distance, your heart rate, and your perceived exertion at the end of the five minutes of brisk exercise.

Repeat the test after several weeks of exercise. There may be a change in as little as four weeks. However, it often takes eight to twelve weeks to see improvement.

Goal: To cover more distance *or* to lower your heart rate *or* to lower your perceived exertion.

Test 2. Time Test

Measure a given distance you intend to walk, bike, or swim. Estimate how far you think you can go in about five minutes. You can pick a number of blocks, an actual distance measured in feet, or lengths in a pool.

Spend three to five minutes warming up. Then, start timing and start moving steadily, briskly, and comfortably. At the finish, record how long it took you to cover your course, your heart rate, and your perceived exertion.

Repeat after several weeks of exercise. You may see changes in as soon as four weeks. However, it often takes eight to twelve weeks for improvement.

Goal: To complete the course in less time *or* to lower your heart rate *or* to lower your perceived exertion.

REFERENCES

Bates, A., and N. Hanson. *Aquatic Exercise Therapy*. Canada: Swystun & Swystun, 1992.

Francis, P., and L. Francis. *If It Hurts, Don't Do It*. Rocklin, Calif.: Prima Publishing, 1988.

Krasevec, Joseph A., and Diane C. Grimes. *Hydrorobics*. Champaign, Ill.: Leisure Press, 1985.

EXERCISE VIDEOTAPES

Sayce, V., and I. Fraser. *Exercise Can Beat Arthritis*. New York: V.I.E.W. Video, 1990.

University of Missouri Arthritis Rehabilitation Research and Training Center. *Good Moves for Every Body*. MA427 HSC (Attn: Video). Columbia, MO 65212. U.S. $30 ppd.

▼ ▼ ▼ ▼ ▼ ▼ ▼

14. Healthy Eating

HEALTHY eating is important for all people, even though food *alone* cannot cure your arthritis or make you healthy. Health depends on heredity, environment, lifestyle, and the interaction of these factors, as well as the health care you receive. Instead of worrying about which "diet" to try for your arthritis, consider how to begin making changes in specific eating habits. Learning to eat well is more than just eating a variety of foods so your body gets the appropriate amounts of all the nutrients it needs to function properly. It also means maximizing the pleasure and enjoyment of food, while coping with disease symptoms and maintaining a healthy weight.

In this chapter, we discuss some simple ways to begin eating well and enjoy doing so. This includes tips for maintaining a healthy weight, minimizing common problems associated with eating and weight management, and coping with the side effects of some medications. Like any of the other self-management techniques discussed in this book, learning to eat well can help you feel more in control of your arthritis.

WHAT IS HEALTHY EATING?

Anyone can eat for good health. It involves two simple steps. The first is to eat foods from all the food groups every day (see the table "Food Groups"). Each food group provides you with some of the different nutrients your body needs to function well, and the table shows examples of typical "servings" that count toward meeting your requirements. The amounts you should eat depend on your age, sex, body size, and activity level. For this reason, the suggested servings are given within a range.

FOOD GROUPS

FOOD GROUP	EXAMPLES OF TYPICAL "SERVING"	

Grain products
 	
5–12 servings per day
	Bread, 1 slice
	English muffin
	Cold cereal, 1 oz (30 g)
	Hot cereal (3/4 cup
	  or 175 ml)
		Pasta or rice, 1/2 cup
		  (125 ml)
		1/2 roll, bun, muffin,
		  bagel, pita or
		  tortilla

Vegetables and fruit 5–10 servings per day	1 medium-size fruit or vegetable Fresh, frozen or canned vegetables or fruit, 1/2 cup (125 ml) Salad, 1 cup (250 ml) Fruit or vegetable juice, 1/2–3/4 cup (125–175 ml)	

Milk products
 	
2–4 servings per day
	Milk, 1 cup (250 ml)
	Yogurt, 3/4–1 cup (175 g)
	Cheese, 2 slices,
	  1–2 oz (50 g)
		Ice milk or frozen
		  yogurt, 1/2 cup

Meat and meat
  substitutes
 	
2–3 servings per day
	Cooked, lean meat, poultry, or fish, 2–3 oz
	  (50–100 g)
	1–2 eggs
	Cooked, dried peas or beans, 1/2 cup (125 ml)
	2 tablespoons (30 ml) of peanut butter
	Tofu, 1/3 cup (100 g)	

Foods that are often
  higher in fat and
  calories. Use in
  moderation:
	Fats and oils
	Sweets
	Salty snacks
		Alcohol
		Soft drinks
		Condiments (relishes,
		  ketchup, jam, etc.)

If you are eating a variety of foods from the first four groups listed above, chances are you are getting the minerals and vitamins you need. Therefore, supplements may not be necessary and cannot take the place of a good, balanced way of eating. Should you choose to take a supplement, select one that contains 50% to 100% of the recommended daily allowance (or recommended nutrient intake) for the different vitamins and minerals. Examples include Centrum, One-a-day, Unicap, as well as the different generic, store-brand varieties. There is no need to take higher doses or "megadoses" of supplements unless prescribed and supervised by your doctor. Too much of some vitamins and minerals can create more health problems and even some toxic reactions.

The second step to eating well is to eat different foods from within each group every day.

MANAGING A HEALTHY WEIGHT

Achieving and maintaining a healthy weight* is especially important for people with arthritis. Your weight can have a considerable impact on your disease symptoms and your ability to exercise or otherwise manage the disease. Therefore, finding a healthy weight and maintaining it are important parts of the self-management process. But what is a healthy weight?

A healthy weight is *not* an "ideal" weight such as one found in a table. There is no such thing as an "ideal" weight for an individual. The tables of "ideal" weights are only guidelines for weight ranges based on population statistics. They should not be used to determine your specific weight target. Being at a healthy weight does not mean being thin or "skinny" like the popular images portrayed in the media. These body shapes and weights are not realistic for most of us. In fact, being too thin sometimes contributes to health problems.

Rather, a healthy weight is one where you decrease your risk of developing health problems, or further complicating existing ones, and feel better both mentally and physically. Finding a healthy weight depends on several factors: your age, your activity level, how much of your weight is fat, where the fat is on your body, and whether or not you have weight-related medical problems such as high blood pressure or a family history of such problems. You may already be at a healthy weight and need only to maintain it by eating well and staying active. Consider asking your doctor to refer you to a nutritionist for help in determining what a healthy weight is for you, given your condition and treatment needs.

---

*Portions of this chapter have been adapted from two publications: *Thinking About Losing Weight?* (Northern California Regional Health Education Center, Kaiser Permanente Medical Care Program, 1990) and *The Weight Kit* (Stanford Center for Research in Disease Prevention, Health Promotion Resource Center, Stanford University, 1990).

If you are considering a change, ask yourself the following questions.

1. Why Change My Weight?

The reasons for losing or gaining weight are different for each individual. The most obvious reason may be your physical health, but there may also be psychological or emotional reasons for wanting to change. Examine for yourself why you want to change.

For example, changing my weight will help me ...

☐ Lessen my disease symptoms (pain, fatigue, depression, etc.).
☐ Give me more energy to do the things I want to do (exercise, hobbies, etc.).
☐ Feel better about myself.
☐ Feel more in control of my disease and/or my life.

If you have other reasons, jot them down here:

_____

_____

2. What Will I Have to Change?

Two ingredients for successful weight management are developing an active lifestyle and making changes in your eating patterns. Let's look closely at what each of these involves.

An active lifestyle involves physical activity, which burns calories and regulates appetite and metabolism, both important for weight management. Physical activity can also help you develop more strength and stamina, as well as move and breathe more easily. In other words, activity doesn't wear you down or out, but actually boosts your energy level. You will find more information about this and tips for choosing activities that suit your needs and lifestyle in Chapters 8–10.

While many people are concerned with losing weight and keeping it off, some people with arthritis struggle to gain and maintain a healthy weight. If you experience a continual or extreme weight loss because your disease or medications interfere with your appetite and/or deplete your body of valuable nutrients (such as proteins, vitamins, and minerals), you may need to work at gaining weight.

Making changes in your eating patterns starts with making small, gradual changes in what you eat. This may mean changing the types or quantity of foods you eat. For example, begin by reducing the fat and increasing the fiber content in the foods you select. Foods that are high in fiber and low in fat help with weight management, but also reduce cholesterol, and prevent constipation and some forms of cancer. The list of "Food Choices" (below) has hints for reducing fat and increasing fiber in your diet. You can find additional information on healthy eating in the references listed at the end of this chapter.

It's best to change gradually. If you increase the amount of fiber you eat too quickly, you may overwhelm your digestive system, experience problems with gas, or become very uncomfortable or constipated. To prevent constipation follow the tips that start on page 218.

Some foods within each group are better sources of a nutrient than others, so by eating a variety of foods from each group, you increase your chances of getting all the nutrients you need. When making these food choices, you should consider emphasizing foods that are high in fiber and low in fat. Below are some tips for doing this.

FOOD CHOICES

HINTS FOR INCREASING FIBER

- ▼ Eat a variety of fruits and vegetables, raw or slightly cooked (steamed).
- ▼ Eat low-fat whole-grain products, including breads, hot or cold cereals, crackers, and brown rice and other whole grains.
- ▼ Drink plenty of water to help move the fiber through.
- ▼ Try cooked dried beans, peas, and lentils as a substitute for meat, for example, baked beans, or split-pea or lentil soup.

HINTS FOR REDUCING FAT

- ▼ Eat moderate-size portions of meat, poultry and fish, 2–3 oz (50-100 g), the size of a deck of cards.
- ▼ Choose leaner cuts of meat.
- ▼ Trim off fat and remove the skin from poultry.
- ▼ Make moderate use of organ meats (liver, kidneys, etc.) and egg yolks.
- ▼ Broil, barbecue, or roast meats instead of frying them.
- ▼ Skim fat off stews and soups. This is easier if the stew has been refrigerated overnight.
- ▼ Use low- or nonfat (skim) milk and milk products.
- ▼ Use added fats like butter, margarine, oils, gravy, sauces, and salad dressings sparingly in food preparation, no more than 3–4 teaspoons (15-20 ml) per day.

▼ Snack on fruit or nonfat yogurt, instead of on cookies or ice cream.

We discuss the specific problems people commonly have to solve while losing, gaining, and maintaining weight, starting on page 177.

3. Am I Ready to Change?

If you have decided that you want to change, next consider if you are ready to make these changes. Success is important. If you are not ready, you may be setting yourself up for failure and those nasty weight "ups and downs." This is not only discouraging but unhealthy. Therefore, try to plan ahead. Is there someone or something that will make it easier for you to change? Or, are there problems or obstacles that will keep you from becoming more active or changing the way you eat? Will worries or concerns about family, friends, work, or other commitments affect your ability to carry out your plans successfully? Looking ahead at these factors can help you find ways to build support for desired changes, as well as minimize possible problems you may encounter along the way. Use the chart on page 175 to identify some factors that you must take into account.

After you have examined these lists, you may find that now is not the right time to start anything. If it is not, set a date in the future for a time when you will reevaluate these changes again. In the meantime, accept that this is the right decision for you at this time, and focus your attention on other goals.

If you decide that now is the right time, start by changing those things that feel most comfortable to you. You don't have to do it all right away. Slow and steady wins the race.

To help get started, keep track of what you are currently doing. For example, write down your daily routine to identify where you might be able to add some exercise. Or keep a food diary for a week to see what and how much you eat, how it's prepared, when and why you are eating. This can help you identify how and where to make changes in your eating patterns, as well as how to shop for and prepare your meals. Next, choose only one or two things to change first. For example, if you find you are eating red meat three or four times per week and you tend to fry it, you may want to try broiling it instead. Or you might buy leaner cuts of meat and substitute fish or poultry for some meals. After you have allowed yourself time to get used to these changes, you can then add more changes. The goal-setting and contracting skills discussed in Chapter 7 can help you do this.

FACTORS INFLUENCING CHANGE

THINGS THAT WILL MAKE IT DIFFICULT FOR ME TO CHANGE	THINGS THAT WILL HELP ME MAKE CHANGES
Example: The holidays are coming up, and there are too many gatherings to prepare for.	Example: I have the support of family and friends.

COMMON PROBLEMS WITH EATING FOR HEALTH

"I enjoy eating out (or I hate to cook), so how do I know if I'm eating well?"

Whether it's because you don't have time, you hate to cook, or you just don't have the energy to go grocery shopping and prepare meals, eating out may suit your needs. This is not necessarily bad if you know which choices are healthy ones.

TIPS ON EATING OUT

▼ Select restaurants that offer variety and flexibility in types of food and methods of preparation. Feel free to ask what is in a dish and how it is prepared, especially if you are eating in a restaurant where the dishes are new or different from what you are used to.

▼ Plan what type of food you will eat and how much. (You can bring the leftovers home.)

▼ Choose items low in fat, sodium, and sugar or ask if they can be prepared that way. For example, appetizers might include steamed seafood or raw vegetables without fancy sauces or dips, or bread without butter. You may request salad with dressing on the side, or bring your own oil-free dress-ing. For an entree, try broiled, barbecued, baked, or steamed dishes. Choose fish or poultry over red meat. Avoid breaded, fried, sauteed or creamy dishes, and choose dishes whose ingredients are listed. Instead of a whole dinner, consider ordering à la carte and lots of vegetables (with-out butter or sauces, of course). For dessert, select fruit, nonfat yogurt, or sherbet. You might even split an entree and a dessert with someone else.

▼ Order first so you aren't tempted to change your order after hearing what others have selected.

▼ If you want fast food, choose salads with dressing on the side, baked pota-toes instead of fries, juice or milk instead of soda, and frozen yogurt instead of ice cream sundaes or shakes.

"I snack while I watch TV (or read)."

If you know this is a problem for you, plan ahead by preparing healthier snacks. For example, rather than eating junk food like chips and cookies, munch on fresh fruit, raw vegetables, or air-popped popcorn. Try designating specific areas at home and work as eating areas and limit your eating to those areas.

"I eat when I'm bored/depressed/feeling lonely."

Many people find comfort in food. Some people eat when they don't have anything else to do or just to fill in time. Some eat when they're feeling down or bothered. Unfortunately, at these times you often lose track of what and how much you eat. These are also the times when celery sticks, apples, or popcorn never seem to do the trick. Instead, you start out with a full bag of potato chips and, by the end of an hour, have only crumbs left. To help control these urges, try to:

▼ Keep a food-mood diary. Every day, list what, how much, and when you eat. Note how you are feeling when you have the urge to eat. Try to spot patterns so you can anticipate when you will want to eat without really being hungry.

▼ Make a plan for when these situations arise. If you catch yourself feeling bored, go for a short walk, work on a jigsaw puzzle, or otherwise occupy your mind and hands. This may be a time to practice a new distraction technique! (Distraction is discussed more in Chapter 15.)

"Healthy food doesn't taste the same as 'real food.' When I eat, I want something with substance, like meat and potatoes! The healthy stuff just doesn't fill me up!"

Just because you are trying to make healthier food choices does not mean that you will never again eat meat and potatoes. It only means that you will change some of the ways you prepare these foods, as well as what you buy at the store. There are also many excellent books that offer tasty and healthy, low-fat recipes. Additional information is available in the references at the end of this chapter.

"But I LOVE to cook!"

If you love to cook, you are in luck. This is your opportunity to take a new cooking class or to buy a new recipe book on healthy cooking. Experiment with different ways to modify your favorite recipes, making them lower in fat, sugar, and sodium. Again, some of the books listed at the end of this chapter may be helpful.

"I'm living alone now, and I'm not used to cooking for one. I find myself overeating so food isn't wasted."

This can be a problem, especially if you are not used to measuring ingredients. You may be overeating or eating a "second dinner" to fill time. Or maybe you are one of those people who will eat for as long as the food is in front of you. Whatever the reason, here are some ways to deal with the extra food:

▼ Don't put the serving dishes on the table. Take as much as you feel you can comfortably eat and bring only your plate to the table.

▼ As soon as you've finished eating, wrap up what you haven't eaten and put it in the refrigerator or freezer. This way you have leftovers for the next day or whenever you don't feel like cooking.

▼ Invite friends over for dinner once in a while, so you can share food and each other's company or plan a potluck supper with neighbors or relatives.

▼ Join a community kitchen or attend a community or church supper.

COMMON PROBLEMS WITH LOSING WEIGHT

"Gosh, I wish I could lose ten pounds in the next two weeks. I want to look good for …"

Sound familiar? Most everyone who has tried to lose weight wants to lose it quickly. This is a hard pattern to break because, although it may be possible to lose five or ten pounds (two to five kg) in one or two weeks, it is not healthy nor is the weight likely to stay off. Rapid weight loss is usually water loss, which can be dangerous, causing the body to become dehydrated. When this happens you may also experience other symptoms such as light-headedness, headaches, fatigue, and poor sleep. Rather than doing this to yourself, try a different approach—one employing realistic goal setting and positive self-talk. (These are discussed in greater detail in Chapters 7 and 15, respectively.) Here are some approaches to sensible weight loss.

▼ Set your goal to lose weight gradually, just one or two pounds (one kg) a month.

▼ Identify the specific steps you will take to lose this weight (for example, increasing activities and/or changing what you eat).

▼ Change your self-talk from "I really need to lose ten pounds right away" to "Losing this weight gradually will help me keep it off for good."

▼ Be patient. You didn't gain weight overnight, so you can't expect to lose it overnight.

"I can lose the first several pounds relatively painlessly, but I just can't seem to lose those last few pounds."

This can be frustrating and puzzling, especially when you have been eating well and staying active. However, it is quite common and usually means that your body has adapted to your new calorie intake and activity levels. While your first impulse may be to cut your calorie intake even further, it probably won't help and could be unhealthy. You want to make changes you can live with.

Ask yourself how much of a difference one, two, or even five pounds will really make. If you are feeling good, chances are you don't need to lose more weight. It is not unhealthy to live with a few extra pounds, if you are staying active and eating low-fat foods. You may already be at a healthy weight given your body size and shape. You may be replacing fat with muscle, which weighs more.

However, if you decide that these pounds must go, try the following:

▼ Modify your goal so you maintain your weight for a few weeks, then try to lose a pound more gradually over the next few weeks.

▼ Try adding to your physical activity or exercise goals, especially if your current activities or exercises have become easy. Increasing your activity level will help you to use more calories and maintain your muscle mass. Less weight will be stored in the form of fat. (Tips for safely increasing your exercise are found in Chapters 10 to 13.)

▼ Again, be patient and allow your body time to adjust to your new patterns.

"I feel so deprived of the foods I love when I try to lose weight."

The key to reaching and maintaining a healthy weight is to make changes you can tolerate, even enjoy. This means they must suit your lifestyle and needs. Unfortunately, when thinking about losing weight, most of us tend to think of all the things we *can't* eat. Change this way of thinking now! There are probably as many (if not more) foods you *can* eat than ones you should limit. Sometimes it is just a matter of learning to prepare foods differently, rather than eliminating them completely. If you like to cook, this is your opportunity to become creative, learning new recipes or finding ways to change old ones. There are many good cookbooks on the market today to help you make this process more enjoyable. Some of these tips were outlined on pages 173-174, and more can be found in the references listed at the end of the chapter.

"I finish eating before everyone and find myself reaching for seconds."

Eating too fast happens for a couple of reasons. One may be that you are limiting yourself to only two or three meals a day, not eating or drinking between meals. This can leave you so hungry at mealtime that you practically inhale your food. Another reason may be that you have not had a chance to slow down and relax before eating. Slowing down your eating can help you decrease your food intake. If you find you are too hungry, feeling stressed out, or in a hurry, try one or more of the following:

▼ Try not to skip meals. In this way you are less likely to overeat at the next meal.

▼ Allow yourself to snack on healthy foods between meals. In fact, plan your snacks for midmorning and afternoon. Keep a banana, some raw vegetables, or a few crackers with you for those "snack attacks."

▼ Eat more frequent, smaller meals. This may also be easier on your digestive system, which won't be overwhelmed by a large meal eaten in a hurry.

▼ Chew your food well. Food is an enjoyable necessity! Chewing your food well also eases the burden on your digestive system.

▼ Drink plenty of water! Six to eight glasses of water per day is recommended. This helps you to eat less, and helps prevent medication side effects, aids elimination, and keeps the kidneys functioning properly.

▼ Try a relaxation method about a half an hour before you eat. Several methods are discussed in Chapter 15.

"I can't do it on my own."

Losing weight isn't easy, but it can be done. Sometimes you just need outside support. For help, you can contact any of the following sources:

▼ A professional nutritionist, through your health plan or local hospital.

▼ A support group such as Weight Watchers or Take Off Pounds Sensibly (TOPS), where you can meet other people who are trying to lose weight or maintain a proper weight.

▼ A weight-reduction course offered by your local health department, your hospital, the community schools, or even your employer.

Another motivation to lose weight, if you are over your proper weight, is that losing pounds can help to relieve pains in your lower joints. This is one case where losing is winning.

COMMON PROBLEMS WITH GAINING WEIGHT

"I don't know how to add pounds."

Here are some ways to increase the amount of calories and/or nutrients you eat. Unfortunately, these may also add some fat to your diet. Check with your doctor or dietitian to see which of the following tips are appropriate for you:

▼ Eat smaller meals frequently during the day.

▼ Snack on calorie-rich foods such as nuts, seeds, and dried fruits.

▼ Drink high-calorie beverages such as shakes and malts.

▼ Eat high protein foods.

▼ Use milk to prepare creamed dishes with meat, fish, or poultry.

▼ Add meat to salads, soups, and casseroles.

▼ Add milk or milk powder to sauces, gravies, cereals, soups, and casseroles.

- Use melted cheese on vegetables and other dishes.

- Add butter, margarine, oils, and cream to dishes.

- Don't skip meals.

- Use protein, vitamin, and mineral supplements if needed.

"Food doesn't taste as good as before."

If you are taking certain medications, you may have noticed a decrease in your taste sensations. To compensate, you may have also noticed that you've been increasing the amount of salt you add to your foods. Be careful because a high sodium intake can cause water retention or bloating, which can result in increased blood pressure. To avoid this, try enhancing the flavors of foods by

- Experimenting with lemon juice, herbs, spices, and other seasonings. Start with just about ¼ teaspoon (5 ml) in a dish for four people.

- Modifying recipes to include a wide variety of ingredients to make the food look and taste more appealing.

- Chewing your food well. This will allow the food to remain in your mouth longer and provide more stimulation to your taste buds.

If the decline in taste is keeping you from getting essential nutrients, you may need to adjust the caloric content of these foods. Tips for doing this are mentioned above.

"By the time I prepare a meal, I'm too tired to eat."

If this is a problem for you, then it's time to develop a plan because you need to eat to maintain your energy level. Here are some hints to help:

- Plan your meals for the week.

- Then go to the grocery store and buy everything you will need.

- Break your food preparation into steps, resting in between.

- Cook enough for two, three, or even more servings, especially if it's something you really like.

- Freeze the extra portions in single-serving sizes. On the days when you are really tired, thaw and reheat one of these precooked, frozen meals.

- Ask for help, especially for those big meals or at family gatherings.

"Sometimes eating causes discomfort." Or, "I really have no appetite."

People who find it difficult, unpleasant, or physically uncomfortable to eat naturally tend to eat less and may be underweight. For some, eating a large meal causes indigestion, discomfort, or nausea. If any of these is a problem for you,

▼ Try eating four to six smaller meals a day, rather than the usual three larger meals.

▼ Avoid foods that produce gas or make you feel bloated. You can determine which affect you this way by trying different foods and observing the results. Often these foods include vegetables such as cabbage, broccoli, brussels sprouts, varieties of onions, beans, and fruits like raw apples, melons, and avocados, especially if eaten in large quantities.

▼ Eat slowly, taking small bites and chewing your food well. You should also pause occasionally during a meal.

▼ Practice a relaxation exercise about half an hour before mealtime, or take time out for a few deep breaths during the meal.

"I can't eat much in one sitting."

There is no real need to eat only three meals a day. In fact, for many it is recommended to eat four to six smaller meals. If you choose to do this, include "no-fuss," high-calorie snacks like milk, bread, and fruits or liquid protein shakes as part of these extra meals. If you still can't finish a whole meal, be sure to eat the portion of your meal that is highest in calories first. Save the vegetables, fruits, and beverages for last.

COMMON PROBLEMS WITH MAINTAINING YOUR WEIGHT

"I've been on a lot of diets before and lost a lot of weight. But I've always gained it back, and then some. It's so frustrating, and I just don't understand why this happens!"

Many of us have experienced this problem; it occurs because the diet was short term and calorie-restricted and did not emphasize changes in eating habits. In fact, this is the problem with many so-called "diets": They involve drastic changes in both what we eat and the way we eat so that they cannot be tolerated for long. Because your body does not know when more food will be available again, it reacts physiologically to this deprivation, slowing its metabolism to adapt to a smaller amount of food energy. Then, when you've had enough of the diet, or have lost the weight and return to your old eating habits, you gain the weight back. Sometimes you even gain back more weight than you lost. Again, the body is responding physiologically, replenishing its stores, usually in the form of fat. This fat serves as a concentrated energy source to be called upon again when calories are restricted. Therefore, the weight goes up and down in cycles, which is both unhealthy and very discouraging.

This situation is further complicated by feelings of deprivation, as you probably had to give up your favorite foods. Therefore, when you reach your goal weight, you begin to eat all of those foods again freely and most likely in larger quantities.

The key to maintaining a healthy weight is developing healthy eating habits that are enjoyable to you and fit into your lifestyle. We have already discussed many of these tips earlier in this chapter. A few additional tips include the following:

▼ Set a small weight range goal that you consider to be healthy for *you*, instead of a specific weight. Weights fluctuate naturally. By setting a range, you will allow yourself some flexibility.

▼ Monitor your activity level. Once you have lost some weight, exercise three to five times a week to improve your chances of keeping the weight off. If possible, gradually increase your activity level.

"I do okay maintaining my weight for a short time. Then something happens beyond my control, and my concerns about what I eat become insignificant. Before I know it I've slipped back into my old eating habits."

If you had only a little slip, don't worry about it. Just continue as if nothing happened. If the slip is longer, try to evaluate why. Is there a situation or circumstance requiring a lot of attention now? If so, weight management may be taking a backseat for a while. This is okay. The sooner you realize this the better, and try to set a date when you will start your weight management program again. You may even want to join a support group and stay with it for at least four to six months. If so, look for one that

▼ Emphasizes good nutrition and the use of a wide variety of foods.

▼ Emphasizes changes in eating habits and patterns.

▼ Gives support in the form of ongoing meetings or long-term follow-up.

ARTHRITIS DIETS AND "CURES"—HOW TO AVOID TRAPS

If you are considering a particular diet (or some other type of alternative treatment) for your arthritis, here are some steps to follow to help you evaluate if it is right for you.

Step 1: Find written information about the diet or treatment that explains how it works and what the proof of effectiveness is.

Step 2: Read the information to determine the type of evidence the author has. Ask yourself: "Is the proof presented as short stories (anecdotes) about individuals or is it based on results from scientific studies (clinical trials)?"

Step 3: If the evidence comes from stories, ask yourself these questions:

▼ Were the people involved different from other people with arthritis or from you in important ways?

▼ Could anything else have caused the results? Were medications or exercise changed along with diet? Could "positive thinking" or a changed outlook have contributed to the results? Could the results have been a coincidence, since arthritis pain tends to come and go over time?

Step 4: If the evidence is based on clinical studies, ask yourself these questions:

▼ Was there a "control" group made up of people similar to the treatment group in most ways, except in that they didn't receive the treatment? Such a group helps sort out the treatment's effects from the other coincidental factors mentioned above.

▼ Were these two groups really similar in age, sex, weight, exercise, and activity patterns and the type and severity of arthritis?

▼ Were the researchers looking for a specific result, which may have biased the way they interpreted or reported the results?

▼ Was the study published in a recent scientific journal where it would have been carefully reviewed by other scientists?

Step 5: If you are still not sure whether or not to try the diet or treatment, talk to your doctor, registered dietitian, nutritionist, or other health professional for advice.

Step 6: If you are unable to talk to any of these health professionals, ask yourself these questions:

▼ Does the "diet" eliminate any of the basic foods or nutrients? If so, you may harm your health if you follow it.

▼ Does the diet stress a few special foods, so that you will have little variety in your meals? Again, if it does, it may harm your health or be too difficult or boring to follow.

▼ Do the foods or supplements cost more than you can afford? If so, following the diet may force you to cut back on or do without other essentials.

▼ Are you willing to put up with the trouble and expense involved, knowing that the chances are your arthritis will *not* be cured?

If you answer no to the first three questions under Step 6 and yes to the last, it probably will not harm you to try the diet (or other treatment) and see if it works for you. Even if it seems to work for you by helping you to manage your weight or other arthritis symptoms, it may not work well for someone else. Eating well, on the other hand, does work for everyone!

To summarize, eating well does not mean that you are forever forbidden to eat certain foods. It means learning to eat a variety of foods in the right quantities to maintain your health and/or better manage your disease symptoms. This involves changing your eating patterns and emphasizing foods that are higher in fiber and lower in fat, sugar, and sodium. These changes are important for effective weight management. If you choose to make some of the changes suggested in this chapter, remember that you should not feel as though you are punishing yourself, nor that this is a life sentence to boring, bland food. As a self-manager, it's up to you to find the changes that are best for you. And if you experience setbacks, identify the problems and work at resolving them. Remember, if you really want to, you can do it!

FOOD AND MEDICATIONS

Food and medicines affect one another. Some drugs used for arthritis are best absorbed when taken on an empty stomach, while others irritate or upset the stomach unless taken with food. Some drugs may even alter your nutritional needs. Therefore, learning how your medicines interact with food can help you prevent some problems with medications.

Whenever you get a new medication, prescription or nonprescription, ask the doctor or pharmacist if you should take it with meals or on an empty stomach. Many of the nonsteroidal, anti-inflammatory drugs (NSAIDs) such as aspirin, Indocin, Clinoril, etc., should be taken with meals and ample fluids to prevent stomach irritation. There is more information about medications and how they should be taken in Chapter 20 of this book.

If your doctor asks you to take a drug with every meal, he or she probably assumes that you eat three meals a day. If you don't, be sure to tell the doctor. You may need different directions for taking your medicines.

The table below discusses some commonly used drugs, their interaction with certain nutrients and the recommended action to take in controlling or preventing problems.

DRUGS AND NUTRITIONAL NEEDS

DRUG	INTERACTION EFFECT	ACTION TO TAKE
Aspirin and other NSAIDs	May cause stomach irritation and bleeding, increasing nutritional needs for iron, vitamin C, and folic acid.	Eat more foods high in iron (meat, legumes, whole-grain products), vitamin C (citrus fruits, dark green vegetables), and folic acid (green leafy vegetables, whole-grain cereals). Check with doctor about need for an iron supplement; this may be preferable to eating larger quantities of meat.

continued

DRUGS AND NUTRITIONAL NEEDS (*continued*)

DRUG	INTERACTION EFFECT	ACTION TO TAKE
Prednisone and other corticosteroids	Cause water retention and increase your need for calcium, potassium, and certain vitamins in order to protect your bones.	Limit salt and sodium based seasonings and sauces added to your food. Avoid foods that taste salty or contain a lot of salt/sodium (including softened water, commercial soups and sauces, and some antacids). Follow nutritional guidelines and eat at least the recommended amounts of meat and milk products. Check with your doctor about calcium, vitamin/mineral supplements.
Antacids	If they contain calcium, antacids can cause constipation. If they contain aluminum, they can interfere with the body's use of phosphorus, a mineral crucial for bone health.	Limit their use and follow the nutritional guidelines in this chapter for preventing constipation and getting recommended amounts of vitamins and minerals. Check with doctor for alternatives.
Laxatives	Laxatives—especially mineral oil, milk of magnesia, and products with phenolphthalein or bisacodyl—reduce the body's ability to absorb nutrients.	Limit their use because they can cause dependency. Try natural methods or products for preventing constipation that are mentioned on page 218.

REFERENCES

General

American Heart Association. *An Active Partnership for the Health of Your Heart.* Dallas: American Heart Association, 1990.

Breitose, P. *Eat Right.* Stanford, Calif.: Stanford Center for Research in Disease Prevention, The Health Promotion Resource Center, Stanford University, 1989.

Breitose, P. *Staying Healthy.* Stanford, Calif.: Stanford Center for Research in Disease Prevention, The Health Promotion Resource Center, Stanford University, 1986.

Breitose, P. *Food for Health.* Stanford, Calif.: Stanford Center for Research in Disease Prevention, The Health Promotion Resource Center, Stanford University, 1982.

Escott-Stump, Sylvia. *Nutrition and Diagnosis-Related Care.* Philadelphia, Pa.: Lea and Febiger, 1988.

Health and Welfare Canada. *Canada's Food Guide to Healthy Eating.* Toronto: Minister of Supply and Services (Cat. No. H39-252/1992E), Canada 1992.

United States Department of Agriculture. *Eating Right the Dietary Guidelines Way.* Hyattsville, Md.: U.S. Department of Agriculture, Human Nutrition Information Service, 1990.

Williams, Sue R. *Essentials of Nutrition and Diet Therapy.* St. Louis, Mo.: Times Mirror/Mosby College Publishing, 1990.

Healthy Recipes

Brody, Jane. *Jane Brody's Good Food Book.* New York: Bantam, 1987.

Clark, M. *Recipes for Your Heart's Delight.* Stanford, Calif.: Stanford Center for Research in Disease Prevention, The Health Promotion Resource Center, Stanford University, 1989.

Lindsay, Anne. *Anne Lindsay's Light Kitchen.* Toronto: Macmillan, 1994.

Schwartz, R. *The Enlightened Eater.* Milwaukee, Wis.: Stoddart Publishing, 1992.

Vegetarian Eating

Lappé, Frances Moore. *Diet for a Small Planet.* New York: Ballantine, 1985.

Robertson, Laurel, Carol Flinders, and Bronwen Godfrey. *Laurel's Kitchen: A Handbook for Vegetarian Cookery and Nutrition.* New York: Bantam, 1978.

Robertson, Laurel, Carol Flinders, and Bronwen Godfrey. *Laurel's Kitchen Recipes.* Berkeley, Calif.: Ten Speed Press, 1993.

Weight Control

Breitrose, P. *The Weight Kit.* Stanford, Calif.: Stanford Center for Research in Disease Prevention, The Health Promotion Resource Center, Stanford University, 1990.

Ferguson, James M. *Learning to Eat: Behavior Modification for Weight Control.* Palo Alto, Calif.: Bull Publishing, 1975.

Nash, Joyce D., and Linda Ormiston. *Taking Charge of Your Weight and Well-Being.* 2nd ed. Palo Alto, Calif.: Bull Publishing, 1989.

Waltz, Julie. *Food Habit Management: A Comprehensive Guide to Dietary Change.* Ed. Fay Ainsworth and Susan Sommerman. Edmonds, Wash.: Northwest Learning Associates, 1982.

▼ ▼ ▼ ▼ ▼ ▼ ▼ ▼ ▼ ▼

PART FIVE

Solving Particular Problems

▼ ▼ ▼ ▼ ▼ ▼ ▼

15. Pain Management

*P*AIN is a problem shared by most people with arthritis. In fact, for many people, it is their number one concern. Unfortunately, pain is a very personal symptom. It cannot be seen by others, and we do not even have good words to describe most pain. Because it is so individual, pain is hard to treat, so it is important for you to know a little about pain.

The pain caused by arthritis really comes from at least three sources.

▼ The disease itself causes pain, from damaged and inflamed joints.

▼ A second type of pain comes from weak, tense muscles. When a joint is damaged, the natural response of the body is to tense the muscles in the area in an effort to protect the joint. Unfortunately, these muscles are often weak from not being used. In addition, tense muscles themselves cause pain by building up lactic acid. Try making a fist and holding it for five minutes to confirm the pain that comes from muscle tension.

▼ A final source of pain is fear and depression. When we are afraid and depressed, everything, including pain, seems worse.

Because pain comes from many sources, pain management must be aimed at all of these sources. The solutions are not found just in this chapter, but throughout the book. For instance, exercise both strengthens muscles and helps them to relax, so an exercise program should be part of your pain management (see Chapters 10–13). Since every excess pound on your body puts several pounds of pressure on your lower joints, one of the best ways to relieve pain in your back, hips, knees, ankles, and feet is to maintain a proper weight (see Chapter 14). A cane or walking stick can also help to relieve hip or knee pain (see page 58). Medication is useful, of course (see Chapter 20). To overcome the fear and depression that aggravate pain, it is important to understand these feelings (see Chapters 17 and 18), to understand the disease, and to become an active arthritis self-manager.

This chapter describes a number of simple pain-management techniques that you can practice almost anytime. Some you may have heard of, such as using heat or cold to reduce pain in particular joints. We also describe cognitive pain-management techniques. These use the mind in different ways to help people to relax their muscles, reduce stress and anxiety, and decrease pain.

All of us at one time or another have experienced the power of the mind and its effect on the body. For example, when we are embarrassed, we might feel flushed and our faces blush. If we think about sucking on a lemon, our mouths pucker and start to water. These simple examples illustrate the ability of our thoughts and feelings to affect our bodies. Therefore, with training and practice you can learn to use your mind effectively to relieve the pain and other symptoms associated with your arthritis. In fact, we know from our experiences with many people that these cognitive techniques are powerful self-management tools. In the following pages we will describe several of these techniques. In order to be able to use them to your best advantage, we suggest you try the following:

1. Read the whole chapter.

2. Try several different techniques. You will probably like some and not others. Be sure you give your chosen technique a fair trial. This means at least two weeks of practice for a minimum of fifteen to twenty minutes a day before you decide if it is going to be helpful.

3. Once you have found two or three techniques you like, think how you will use each one. For example, some exercises can be done anywhere while others require a quiet place. The best pain managers use a variety of techniques that can be mixed and matched to the situations in daily life. Include your choices in your weekly contract.

4. Finally, place some clues in your environment to remind you to practice your pain-management skills. You have to be regular with your program for it to work. For example, place some stars or other stickers where you will see them, and they will remind you to practice your skills. You can put a star on your mirror, your office or home telephone, or the dashboard of your car. Change the stickers every month or so. This will help you notice them.

RELAXATION TECHNIQUES

So much has been said and written about relaxation that most of us are completely confused. It is not a cure-all, but neither is it a hoax. Rather, like most treatment methods, it has specific uses. The advantage of relaxation in the management of arthritis is that muscles become less tense and thus it is easier and less painful to move the joints. In addition to releasing tension throughout the body, relaxation exercises help you sleep, and they are particularly helpful in relieving pain.

Like all exercise, the following techniques take practice. Thus, if you feel you are not accomplishing anything, be patient and keep trying. Try another method if the one you choose does not seem to work for you, but first give it two full weeks trial. Relaxation techniques should be practiced at least fifteen to twenty minutes a day, five days a week.

With many forms of arthritis, it is wise to take short rest periods during the day, to avoid undue fatigue and to relieve stress on the joints. This is an excellent time to practice relaxation techniques.

The following are examples of relaxation techniques. Once you choose the one that works best for you, tape-record the technique. This is not necessary but is sometimes helpful if you find it hard to concentrate. With an inexpensive cassette recorder you can tape a routine to follow so you won't have to think hard or look at this book while you are trying to relax.

Here are some guidelines that will help you practice the relaxation techniques described in this chapter:

1. Pick a quiet time and place where you will not be disturbed for fifteen to twenty minutes.
2. Try to practice daily, but not less than five times a week.
3. Don't expect miracles. It will probably take three to four weeks of practice before you really start to notice benefits.
4. Relaxation should be helpful. At worst, you may find it boring, but if it is unpleasant or makes you nervous, then you might do better with other pain-management techniques.

Jacobson's Progressive Relaxation

Many years ago a physiologist, Edmund Jacobson, discovered that in order to relax one must know what it feels like to be relaxed and to be tense. He believed that if one could recognize tension, one could then let it go and relax. Thus, he designed a very simple set of exercises to assist with the learning process.*

To relax muscles, you need to know how to scan your body, recognize where you are holding tension, and release that tension. The first step is to become familiar with the difference between the feeling of tension and the feeling of relaxation. This brief exercise will allow you to compare those feelings and, with practice, to spot and release tension anywhere in your body.

For just a little while, let go of all outside concerns. Progressive relaxation is best done lying on your back either on a rug or in bed. However, it can be done seated in a comfortable chair. It can even be done while traveling in the car (provided you are not driving at the time), airplane, or train. Choose a quiet time and place where you will not be disturbed for at least fifteen minutes.

Make yourself as comfortable as possible. Uncross your legs, ankles, and arms. Allow your body to feel completely supported by the surface beneath you.

You may want to close your eyes, as a way of closing out any unnecessary distractions.

Begin by taking a deep breath, breathing in through your nose, filling your chest, and breathing all the way down to the abdomen. When you're ready to breathe out, breathe out through pursed lips slowly and completely. As you breathe out, let as much tension as possible flow out with your breath. Let all your muscles feel heavy, and let your whole body just sink into the surface beneath you.

This exercise will guide you through the major muscle groups from your feet to your head, asking you to first tense and then relax those muscles. If you have pain in any part of your body today, don't tense that area. Instead just notice any tension that may already be there and let go of that tension.

Become aware of the muscles of your **feet and calves.** Pull your toes back up toward your knees. Hold your feet in this position ... noticing the sensations.... Now relax your feet and release the tension. Observe any changes in sensations as you let go of the tension.

Now tighten the large muscles of your **thighs and buttocks.** Hold the muscles tense. And as you do, be aware of the sensations.... And now release

---

*Much of this section has been adapted from Gordon Paul, *Insight vs. Desensitization in Psychotherapy: An Experiment in Anxiety Reduction* (Stanford, Calif.: Stanford University Press, 1966).

these muscles, allowing them to feel soft, as if they're melting into the surface beneath you.

Now turn your attention to your **abdomen and chest**. Tense these muscles by holding in your abdomen and tightening the muscles on your chest wall. Notice a tendency to hold your breath as you tense these muscles. Now release the tension. You may feel a natural desire to take a deep breath to release even more of the tension, and so do that now. Breathe in deeply through your nose, and when you breathe out, allow your abdomen and chest to soften.

Now, stretching your fingers out straight, tighten the muscles of your **hands and arms**. Release and feel the tension flowing out and the circulation returning.

Next press your shoulder blades together, tightening the muscles in your **upper back, shoulders and neck**. This is a place many people carry tension. . . . And relax. You may notice that your muscles feel a little warmer and more alive.

Finally, tighten all the muscles of your **face and head**. . . . Notice the tension around your eyes and in your jaw. Now release the tension, allowing the muscles around your eyes to soften and your mouth to remain slightly open as your jaw relaxes. Notice the difference.

Now take another deep breath, and when you're ready to breathe out, allow any remaining tension to flow out with your breath and your whole body to be even more deeply relaxed.

And now just enjoy this feeling of relaxation for a little while. . . . In this quiet state, notice the heaviness of your muscles . . . and the rhythm of your breathing . . . as you breathe in and breathe out. . . .

Remember this pleasant feeling. You can quiet your mind and body in this way anytime you do this exercise. With practice, you will be able to create this feeling just by taking a deep breath.

As you prepare to end this exercise, picture yourself bringing this feeling of quiet and calm to whatever you are going to do next. And then take one more deep breath and, when you're ready, open your eyes.

Body Scan

This is an alternative to the Jacobson technique and does not require any movement. Like Jacobson, it is best done on your back, but can be done in any comfortable position. First, you must become aware of your breathing.

Spend a few minutes concentrating on your breath as it enters and leaves your body. Try directing your breath to your belly or abdomen. This is called diaphragmatic breathing and is important for all kinds of relaxation.

After three or four minutes of concentrating on your breathing, move your attention to your toes. Don't move your toes, just think about how they feel. Don't worry if you don't feel anything at all. If you find any tension, let it go as you breathe out.

After a few moments of concentrating on your toes, change your attention to the bottom of your feet. Again, don't move, just concentrate on any sensations you have. Let go of any tension you may find as you breathe out. Next concentrate on the top of your feet and your ankles. After a few more moments shift your attention to your lower legs.

Continue this process, shifting your attention every few moments to another portion of the body, working slowly upward. If you find tension, let it go as you breathe out. If at any time your mind wanders, bring your attention back to the feelings in your body and to your breathing.

This technique can also be used for getting back to sleep, as it helps to clear your mind of worries and/or other distracting thoughts. The secret is to give full attention to the body scan.

BREATHING EXERCISES

These are really a special form of relaxation. You should concentrate on your breathing, taking a long slow breath through your nose, holding it for a few seconds, and breathing out through your mouth. As you do this, say "relax" to yourself. You can try to focus the breath either at the back of your chest or, if you wish, on your painful joint. The most important thing is to concentrate on your breathing and keep it slow and easy. To check this, you might place a lit candle in front of you. When blowing out a breath, you should make the candle flicker but not go out.

One problem with breathing exercises is that sometimes people hyperventilate. That is, they have a hard time catching their breath. Hyperventilation is scary but not dangerous. Strangely enough, it is caused by having too much oxygen and not enough carbon dioxide. An easy way to restore the balance is to breathe into a closed paper bag for a short time. Better yet, don't hyperventilate. By keeping your breathing slow and easy, you can completely avoid this problem.

The Relaxation Response

During the early 1970s Dr. Herbert Benson did extensive work on what he calls the relaxation response. He says that our bodies have several natural states. For example, if you meet a lion on the street, you will probably become quite tense—your response will be a "fight-or-flight" response. After extreme tension, the body's natural response is to relax. This is what happens after a sexual climax. As life becomes more and more complex, our bodies tend to stay in a constant state of tension. Thus, to elicit the relaxation response, many people will consciously need to practice the following exercise.

Four Basic Elements

1. **A quiet environment.** Turn off internal stimuli and external distractions.
2. **An object to dwell upon, or a mental device.** For example, repeat a word or sound like the word one, gaze at a symbol like a flower, or concentrate on a feeling such as peace.
3. **A passive attitude.** This is the most essential factor. It is an emptying of all thoughts and distractions from your mind. Thoughts, imagery, and feelings may drift into awareness—don't concentrate on them, just allow them to pass on.
4. **A comfortable position.** You should be comfortable enough to remain in the same position for twenty minutes.

Technique for Eliciting the Relaxation Response

1. Sit quietly in a comfortable position.
2. Close your eyes.
3. Deeply relax all your muscles, beginning at your feet and progressing up to your face. Keep them relaxed. If you wish, you can use the Body Scan just described.
4. Breathe in through your nose. Become aware of your breathing. As you breathe out through your mouth, say the word *one* silently to yourself. Try to empty all thoughts from your mind; concentrate on *one*.
5. Continue for ten to twenty minutes—you may open your eyes to check the time, but do not use an alarm. When you finish, sit quietly for several minutes, at first with your eyes closed. Do not stand up for a few minutes.
6. Do not worry about whether you are successful in achieving a deep level of relaxation. Maintain a passive attitude and permit relaxation to occur at its own pace. When distracting thoughts occur, try to ignore them by not dwelling upon them, and return to repeating *one*.

7. Practice once or twice daily, but ideally not within two hours after any meal, since digestive processes seem to interfere with the relaxation responses.

You may have noticed that this exercise is very much like meditation. In fact, meditation has provided the principles of the relaxation response. There is no need to spend several hundred dollars to learn to meditate. You now know all the steps.

Guided Imagery

Another technique is called guided imagery. This is like a guided daydream where you transport yourself to another time and place. It is as though you were taking a mental stroll. The guided imagery script presented here can be used in several different ways, depending on what technique works best for you. Consider each of the following:

1. Read the script over several times to familiarize yourself with it. Then sit or lie in a quiet place and try to reconstruct the scene in your mind. The script should take ten to fifteen minutes to complete.
2. Have a family member or friend slowly read you the script. Wherever there is a series of dots (…) he or she should pause for at least ten seconds.
3. Make a tape of the script and play it to yourself.

"A Walk in the Country"

You're giving yourself some time to quiet your mind and body. Allow yourself to settle comfortably, wherever you are right now. If you wish, you can close your eyes. Breathe in deeply, through your nose, expanding your abdomen and filling your lungs. Pursing your lips, exhale through your mouth slowly and completely, allowing your body to sink heavily into the surface beneath you. … And once again breathe in through your nose and all the way down to your abdomen, and then breathe out slowly through pursed lips—letting go of tension, letting go of anything that's on your mind right now and just allowing yourself to be present in this moment. …

Imagine yourself walking along a peaceful old country road. The sun is warm on your back … the birds are singing … the air is calm and fragrant.

As you walk along, your mind naturally wanders to the concerns and worries of the day. Then you come upon a box by the side of the road and

---

it occurs to you that this box is a perfect place to leave your cares behind while you enjoy this time in the country. So you open the box and put into it any concerns, worries, or pressures that you're carrying with you. You close the box and fasten it securely, knowing that you can come back and deal with those concerns whenever you're ready.

You feel lighter as you progress down the road. Soon you come across an old gate. The gate creaks as you open it and go through.

You find yourself in an overgrown garden—flowers growing where they've seeded themselves, vines climbing over a fallen tree, soft green wild grasses, and shade trees.

Breathe deeply, smelling the flowers ... listen to the birds and insects ... feel the gentle breeze warm against your skin. All of your senses are alive and responding with pleasure to this peaceful time and place.

When you're ready to move on, you leisurely follow a path behind the garden, eventually coming to a more wooded area. As you enter this area, your eyes find the trees and plantlife restful to look on. The sun is filtered through the leaves. The air feels mild and a little cooler. You become aware of the sound and fragrance of a nearby stream. You pause and take in the sights and sounds, breathing deeply of the cool and fragrant air several times. . . . And with each breath, you feel more refreshed.

Continuing along the path for a while, you come to the stream. It's clear and clean as it flows and tumbles over the rocks and some fallen logs. You follow the path along the creek for a way, and after a while, you come out into a sunlit clearing, where you discover a small waterfall emptying into a quiet pool of water.

You find a comfortable place to sit for a while, a perfect spot where you can feel completely relaxed.

You feel good as you allow yourself to just enjoy the warmth and solitude of this peaceful place.

After a while, you become aware that it is time to return. You arise and walk back down the path, through the cool and fragrant trees, out into the sun-drenched overgrown garden. . . . One last smell of the flowers, and out the creaky gate.

You leave this country retreat for now and return down the road. You notice you feel calm and rested. You know that you can visit this special place whenever you wish to take some time to refresh yourself and renew your energy.

Vivid Imagery

This is a little like guided imagery but can be used for longer periods or while you are engaged in other activities.

One way to use imagery is to recall pleasant scenes from your past. For example, try to remember every detail of a special holiday or party that made you happy. Who was there? What happened? What did you talk about? Of course, you can do the same sort of thing with a vacation. Another way to use imagery is to fill in the details of a pleasant fantasy. How would you spend a million dollars? What would be your ideal romantic encounter? What would your ideal home or garden be like?

Sometimes warm imagery can be especially helpful, such as thinking of yourself on a warm beach or visiting a tropical island. On the other hand, if you live somewhere that is very warm, cool imagery such as a forest or shaded path may be more relaxing.

Another form of vivid imagery is to think of symbols that represent painful parts of your body. For example, a painful joint might be red or might have a tight band around it or even a lion biting it.

Now try to change the image. Make the red fade until there is no color left, or imagine the band stretching and stretching until it falls off. Change the lion into a purring kitten.

A final way to use vivid imagery is to help you with goal setting (see Chapter 7). After you set your weekly contract, take a few minutes to imagine yourself taking a walk, doing your exercises, or taking your medications. Studies have shown that these few minutes of imagery will help you accomplish your goal. Many people become very skilled at vivid imagery. They find that as they change their pain images, the pain decreases.

DISSOCIATION

This technique involves mentally separating yourself from the painful part of your body. It is especially effective when pain is so severe that it is impossible to distract yourself.

To use dissociation, picture that the painful part of your body is separate from the rest of your body. Imagine that this body part is completely insensitive and therefore does not feel any pain. For example, tell yourself that your joint does not belong to you; it is completely separate from you. You cannot feel anything that happens to it. Whatever happens to your joint does not affect you at all. You can even imagine that you have floated away from your body and are looking at it from across the room.

DISTRACTION

Because our minds have trouble focusing on more than one thing at a time, you can lessen pain by focusing on something else. This technique can be especially helpful if you are going to do some short activity you know to be painful, such as climbing stairs or opening a jar. Following are some suggestions for practicing distraction, also called "attention refocusing."

▼ While climbing stairs, plan exactly what you will be doing when you get to the top. Be as detailed as possible. Or you might name a different bird or flower for each step. You can even try to visualize a bird or flower for every letter of the alphabet.

▼ During any painful activity, think of a person's name, a bird, a food, or whatever, for every letter of the alphabet. If you get stuck on one letter, go on to the next. (This is also a good exercise if you have problems sleeping.)

▼ While sweeping, vacuuming, or mopping, imagine that the floor is a map of North America. Try to name all the states and provinces going from east to west or north to south. You can also do this with the map of Europe or, if you are really good in geography, Africa. If geography is not your strong suit, think of your favorite store and where each department is located.

▼ When getting up from a chair or out of a car, imagine that you are in a spaceship where you are almost weightless, floating effortlessly upward. Or, try counting backward from one thousand by threes, each time getting as far as you can until you are standing. Try to break your old record.

▼ While opening a jar, think of as many uses as you can for the jar. Or try to remember the words of a song and imagine the story taking place inside the jar. There are, of course, a million variations, now that you have the refocusing idea.

So far we have discussed short-term distraction techniques that involve using the mind. Distraction also works well for longer activities or projects, or when the pain tends to last longer. In these cases, the mind is not focused internally, but rather externally on some type of activity. For example, if you have continual pain or are feeling slightly depressed, find an activity that interests and distracts you from the problem. The activity can be almost anything, from gardening to cooking, reading, going to a movie or even doing volunteer work. A mark of a successful self-manager is that he or she has a variety of interests and always seems to be doing something.

RELABELING

This technique is the opposite of distraction or attention refocusing. Rather than thinking of something else, you will think about your pain. However, you will do more than that. You will analyze the pain. Is it sharp, dull, hot, cold? Exactly what are the sensations that you are feeling? Now, concentrate on your pulse, or the muscle tension in or around your joint, but don't think of "pain." Think of the various sensations. These sensations may increase, decrease, or level off. Just go along with them. See if you can begin to think of the sensations as mere dullness, as if the joint had become completely numb.

PRAYER

Over the years, we have had many people tell us that prayer has been very helpful in managing their pain. In many ways, prayer is similar to some relaxation techniques, and in other ways, it may be a dissociation technique. However, one does not need to have a scientific rationale for everything. As the oldest of all pain-management techniques, prayer is very important for many successful arthritis pain managers.

SELF-TALK: "I KNOW I CAN"

All of us talk to ourselves all the time. For example, when waking up in the morning, we think, "I really don't want to get out of bed. I'm tired and don't want to go to work today." Or at the end of an enjoyable evening we think, "Gee, that was really fun. I should get out more often." These things we think or say to ourselves are referred to as "self-talk."

All of our self-talk is learned from others and becomes a part of us as we grow up. It comes in many forms, mostly negative. Negative self-statements are usually in the form of phrases that begin like these: "I just can't do ..." "If only I could or didn't ..." "I just don't have the energy ..." This type of self-talk reflects the doubts and fears we have about ourselves in general, and about our abilities to deal with arthritis and its symptoms, in particular. In fact, negative self-talk can worsen pain, depression, and fatigue.

What we say to ourselves plays a major role in determining our success or failure in becoming good self-managers. Therefore, learning to make self-talk work *for* you instead of *against* you, by changing those negative statements to positive ones, will help you manage your symptoms more effectively. This change, as with any habit, requires practice and includes the following steps:

1. **Listen carefully to what you say *to* or *about* yourself,** both out loud and silently. Then write down all the negative self-talk statements. Pay special attention to the things you say during times that are particularly difficult for you. For example, what do you say to yourself when getting up in the morning with pain, while doing those exercises you don't really like, or at those times when you are feeling blue?

2. **Work on replacing each negative statement** you identified with a positive one, and write these down. Positive statements should reflect the better you, and your decision to be in control. For example, negative statements such as "I don't want to get up," "I'm too tired and I hurt," "I can't do the things I like anymore so why bother," or "I'm good for nothing," become positive messages, such as "I have the energy to get up and do the things I enjoy," or "I know I can do anything I believe I can," "People like me and I feel good about myself," or "Other people need and depend on me; I'm worthwhile."

3. **Read and rehearse these positive statements,** mentally or with another person. It is this conscious repetition or memorization of the positive statements that will help you replace those old, habitual negative statements.

4. **Practice these new statements in real situations.** This practice, along with time and patience, will help the new patterns of thinking become automatic.

Once established, positive self-talk can be a powerful self-management tool that can help you cope better with specific symptoms, as well as master some of the other skills discussed in this book.

As with exercise and other acquired skills, using your mind to manage your arthritis requires both practice and time before you'll begin to notice the benefits. Therefore, if you feel like you are not accomplishing anything, don't give up. Be patient and keep on trying.

HEAT AND COLD

Sometimes pain can be decreased by stimulating the skin over the painful area. This stimulation can be done with heat, such as a hot pad or a warm bath or shower (directed at the sore area). Some people prefer cold for soothing pain. A bag of frozen peas or corn makes an inexpensive, reusable ice pack. Whether using heat or cold, do it for fifteen to twenty minutes.

Another way to stimulate the skin is by using a counterirritant such as any of the mentholated creams, which give a cooling effect.

MASSAGE

Many people find that massage or rubbing the painful area can be very helpful. Massage is actually one of the oldest forms of pain management for arthritis. Hippocrates (c. 460–380 B.C.) said that "physicians must be experienced in many things, but assuredly also in rubbing that can bind a joint that is loose and loosen a joint that is too hard." Self-massage is a simple procedure that can be performed with little practice or preparation. It stimulates the skin, underlying tissues, and muscles by means of applied pressure and stretching.

Massage is not appropriate on a "hot joint," an infected joint, or one that is suffering from phlebitis, thrombophlebitis, or skin eruptions. Following are some basic massage techniques. A little experience will help you decide which works best for you.

After any kind of self-massage, allow yourself a minute to relax and let the tension subside. Breath deeply.

Stroking

Fit your hand to the contour of the muscle you want to massage and move it over the skin. By slightly cupping the hand, the palm and fingers will glide firmly over the muscle. A slow rhythmic movement repeated over the tense or sore area works best. Experiment with different pressures.

Kneading

If you have ever reached up and squeezed your tense neck or shoulder muscles, you were kneading. As if you are kneading dough, grasp the muscle between the palm and fingers or between the thumb and fingers, then slightly lift and squeeze it. Don't pinch the skin, but work more deeply into the muscle itself. A slow, rhythmic squeeze and release works best. Don't knead one spot for more than fifteen or twenty seconds.

Deep Circular Movement or Friction

To create friction that penetrates into the muscle, make small circular movements with the tips of the fingers, the thumb, or the heel of the hand, depending on how large an area you want to massage. Keeping the fingers, thumb, or palm in one place, begin lightly making small circles and slowly increase the pressure. Don't overdo it. After ten seconds or so, move to another spot and repeat.

A Simple Massage Tool

One way of massaging your back, neck, and shoulders is to put a tennis ball in a sock or stocking. By manipulating the sock up or down, you can place it in the area you wish to massage. Then manipulate the ball between your back and the wall or the back of a chair. Try it. This is much easier than it sounds.

A WORD OF CAUTION

The pain-management techniques taught in this chapter, along with such other techniques as self-hypnosis, biofeedback, and acupressure, are still being studied for their usefulness in managing arthritis. We make no special claims for them. Many people in our classes report substantial benefits from these practices, however, and we feel that they have merit if used as an adjunct to and not a substitute for a basic, sound program that is medically directed.

Hypnosis is generally not recommended for people with arthritis. Like certain narcotics, it can mask pain and may thereby cause you to damage your joints. Some of the techniques discussed in this chapter are similar to those used in *self*-hypnosis, however.

Unfortunately, various pain-management techniques are sold in expensive packages as cure-alls for almost everything. Such expensive courses and treatments are *not* necessary. If you want to further explore these techniques, check the following points first to avoid unnecessary expense and disappointment.

1. Is the course or treatment offered by a reputable institution?
2. Is the cost reasonable? (Ten to fifteen dollars for each hour of small-group instruction is about average in the U.S.)
3. Are claims or promises made for a cure? If so, look elsewhere.

REFERENCES

Benson, Herbert, and Miriam Klipper. *The Relaxation Response.* New York: Avon, 1987.

Lipton, Samuel. *Conquering Pain: How to Overcome the Discomfort of Arthritis, Backache, Heart Disease, Childbirth, Period Pain, and Many Other Common Conditions.* New York: Arco, 1985.

TAPES

Relaxation tapes for people with arthritis are available from the Stanford Arthritis Center. Write to: Stanford Arthritis Center—Tapes, 1000 Welch Road, Suite 204, Palo Alto, CA 94304. (See also page 310.)

Mindful Meditation Practice Tapes with Jon Kabat-Zinn (Series I) are available from: Stress Reduction Tapes, P.O. Box 547, Lexington, MA 02173.

▼ ▼ ▼ ▼ ▼ ▼ ▼

16. Getting a Good Night's Sleep

SLEEP is vital for maintaining a healthy outlook on life. It allows our bodies to heal and our energy to be replenished. As explained in Chapter 5, lack of restful sleep also contributes to fibromyalgia.

BEDS

A comfortable bed that allows ease of movement and good body support is the first requirement for a good night's sleep. This usually means a good-quality firm mattress that supports the spine and does not allow the body to sag in the middle of the bed. A bedboard, made of three-quarter-inch or half-inch (1 or 2 cm) plywood, can be placed between the mattress and the box spring to increase firmness. Bedboards can be bought commercially or constructed at home.

Heated waterbeds or airbeds are helpful for some people with arthritis, because they support weight evenly by conforming to the body's shape. Others find these beds uncomfortable. If you are interested, try one out at a friend's home or a hotel for a few nights to decide if it is right for you.

An electric blanket, used at a low heat, is another effective way of providing heat while sleeping, especially for cool or damp nights. Or you might try an electric or wool mattress pad. If you decide to use one or the other, be sure to follow the instructions carefully.

SLEEPING POSITIONS

The best sleeping position depends on which joints are involved. For most people without arthritis of the knees or hips the best position is sleeping on one's side or back. In either case, it is best to use a small soft pillow to support the curvature of the neck and maintain normal neck alignment. Pillows may also be used under the knees to relieve back pain. However, care should be taken not to maintain this position continuously. If you have knee problems, check with your doctor before using a pillow under your knees even for a short period, as it can cause knee contractures. In the side-lying position, a small pillow can be placed between the knees.

For people with hip or knee problems, the best sleeping position is one where the knees are straight and the hips are in a neutral position (not rotated to the sides). There are also a few dos and don'ts.

▼ Do try to rest on your stomach for ten or fifteen minutes a day. This will help prevent flexion contractures of the hips.

▼ If it does not bother you, try putting a small pillow under your ankles while sleeping on your back. (This will keep your knees straight.)

▼ Don't sleep with pillows under your knees, even if this is more comfortable.

For people with back problems, often a comfortable way to sleep is the side-lying position, in which you lie on your side with knees bent. In this position it can be helpful to place a pillow between the knees to alleviate stress on the hips and lower back. A pillow can also be placed under the upper arm to reduce stress on the shoulder joint. But in most cases, your body will tell you the best position. There is no single right way.

If you have ankylosing spondylitis, there are some specific sleep positions that will help prevent deformity and loss of mobility of the spine. Sleep on your stomach or flat on your back. Avoid using high pillows under your head; sleep without a pillow if possible. Place a small pillow between your shoulder blades when you sleep on your back.

SLEEPING PILLS

Sedatives and sleeping pills should be used with caution. They may be habit-forming, suppress important stages of sleep, and cause depression. They only rarely solve sleep problems; the medication taken to control sleep may actually produce a disturbed night's sleep. This is also true of alcohol. If you are using medications and decide to stop, do so gradually.

Certain types of antidepressant medications can be helpful for sleep that is disturbed by pain. The dosage used is much smaller than that used for depression. These medications do not have the potential addictive side effects that many sedatives and sleeping pills have. Ask your physician about them.

INSOMNIA

There is no known serious complication from lack of sleep. If you go without sleep long enough, you will fall asleep, so don't worry. If you can't sleep, don't lie in bed feeling guilty or bored—get up and do something you enjoy, like reading a book or listening to music, until you are sleepy. You need less sleep as you age, so be sure your insomnia is not due to sleeping too much. People worry more about sleeping problems than they need to.

Still, insomnia is a problem that affects all of us at one time or another. It can be a cause of concern if it occurs frequently and involves recurrent daytime fatigue or depression. The causes of insomnia are many, some of which are feelings of anxiety or worry, pain or discomfort due to a medical condition, or an unfamiliar sleeping environment. Other contributing factors may be improper self-treatment or failure to follow the practitioner's recommended dosage or directions for medications. If your sleeping problem continues, you may want to seek a physician's advice.

Some hints for a more comfortable night's sleep include the following:

▼ Maintain a regular sleep schedule so that you go to bed and awaken at about the same time each night and morning.

▼ For relief of pain and inflammation at night, take aspirin or anti-inflammatory drugs as your doctor prescribes, and be sure to take the proper dose at bedtime. Painkillers should be used with great caution. To maintain a good level of aspirin throughout the night, try time-released aspirin.

▼ Use some of the relaxation techniques described in Chapter 15, or create one of your own that is particularly relaxing to you and will settle the day's thoughts and ease the body's tensions. (Distracting yourself by counting backward from one thousand by twos or threes is especially helpful.)

▼ Wait until you are sleepy and your body is ready and eager to go to sleep; going to bed early to ensure a good night's sleep is often counterproductive.

▼ Avoid caffeine (coffee, tea, soft drinks, chocolate) for several hours before bedtime because it can act as a stimulant.

▼ Moderate your alcohol intake; alcohol may cause an erratic night's sleep and restlessness. Avoid any alcohol for three or four hours before bedtime.

▼ Provide yourself with a comfortable environment. Your environment includes mattress, lighting, noise level, temperature, and ventilation.

▼ Try taking a warm bath (not hot) before going to bed.

▼ Get as much exercise as you can during the day, but refrain from exercising immediately before bedtime.

▼ Don't do things that excite you just before going to sleep.

▼ Avoid naps if you are having problems sleeping at night.

▼ Get used to doing the same things every night before going to bed. By developing a "time-to-get-ready-for-bed" routine, you will be telling your body that it's time to start winding down and relaxing.

If you do wake up with stiffness during the night, try some easier exercises (or small amounts in the pain-free range) right in the bed to reduce discomfort and pain, allowing for a more undisturbed and restful sleep.

REFERENCES

Coleman, Richard M. *Wide Awake at 3:00 AM: By Choice or Chance.* New York: W. H. Freeman, 1986.

Oswald, Ian, and Kristine Adam. *Get a Better Night's Sleep.* North Ryde, NSW Australia: Methuen, 1983.

▼ ▼ ▼ ▼ ▼ ▼ ▼

17. Depression, Fatigue, and Other Symptoms

SOMETIMES people with arthritis suffer from other problems brought on by their pain, by frustration, or even by the arthritis medications they take. These problems, or people's common response to them, can make life much worse than the arthritis alone. In this chapter and the next we deal with several such symptoms, some of which you might not even recognize as being related to arthritis. This chapter covers depression, pain, fatigue, and constipation. Chapter 18 discusses the emotional and interpersonal side of coping with arthritis, including working, talking with loved ones, and remaining intimate.

DEPRESSION

One of the most frequent symptoms associated with arthritis is depression. (Some people prefer to say they are "blue" or "feeling down" instead of "depressed.") Depression and pain and concerns about growing old are often parts of a vicious circle. The more depressed you are, the more pain you feel; the more pain you feel, the more stressed you become. The more stressed you become, the more depressed you are. Depression makes you tired; fatigue aggravates your depression and pain, and so on.

Pain Cycle

Disease Pain

Fatigue

Tense Muscles

Depression

Psychological Stress

We have already discussed a number of ways to deal with pain, including heat, relaxation, and exercise. It is when you are the most depressed that you need to pay the most attention to these techniques. Continue to do these things when you are feeling well in order to maintain your good spirits. Take your medicine and do your exercises—even if you don't feel like it. But you also want to lick the depression that is making everything worse.

It is easy to tell when you have pain. But it is not as easy to recognize when you are depressed. Just as there are many degrees of pain, so there are many different degrees of depression. If your arthritis is a significant problem, you almost certainly have or have had some problems with depression; such problems are normal. Everyone feels depression at some time. It is how you handle it that makes the difference. The following fourteen signs have to do with depression, and you probably have had some of them, in either mild or severe form.

1. Loss of interest in friends or activities. Not being home to friends, perhaps not even answering the doorbell or the telephone.
2. Isolation. Not wanting to talk to anyone, avoiding friends you happen to meet in the street.
3. Difficulty sleeping, changed sleeping patterns, interrupted sleep, or sleeping more than usual. Often, going to sleep easily, but awakening and being unable to return to sleep. (It is important to remember that older people need less sleep.)
4. Change in eating habits, either loss of interest in food or excessive eating.
5. Loss of interest in personal care and grooming.
6. Unintentional weight change, either gain or loss, of more than ten pounds (4 kg) in a short period of time.
7. A general feeling of unhappiness lasting longer than six weeks.
8. Loss of interest in being held or in sex. Intimacy problems can sometimes be due to medications and they are very important, so be sure to talk them over with your doctor. See also page 229.
9. Suicidal thoughts.
10. Frequent accidents. Watch for a pattern of increased carelessness, accidents while walking or driving, dropping things, and so forth.
11. Low self-image. A feeling of worthlessness, a negative image of your body, wondering if it is all worth it.
12. Frequent arguments. A tendency to blow up easily over minor matters, over things that never bothered you before.

13. Loss of energy. Feeling tired all of the time.
14. Inability to make decisions. Feeling confused and unable to concentrate.

If some of these seem familiar, you may well be depressed. There are at least a dozen things you can do to change the situation. But, since you are depressed, you may not feel like making the effort. Force yourself or get someone to help you into action. Find someone to talk with. Here are the twelve actions:

1. If your unhappiness has caused you to think seriously about killing yourself, get some help from your doctor, good friends, a member of the clergy, a psychologist, or a social worker. Call your mental health center, doctor, suicide prevention center, a friend, clerical counselor, or senior center. Do not delay. Arthritis problems are not things to kill yourself over, and these feelings will pass and you will feel better. So get help and don't let a tragedy happen.

2. Are you taking tranquilizers or narcotic painkillers? These include drugs such as Valium, Librium, reserpine, codeine, vicodin, sleeping medications, and other "downers." These drugs intensify depression, and the sooner you can stop taking them, the better you will be. Your depression may well be a drug side effect. If you are not sure what you are taking or what the side effects might be, check with the doctor or pharmacist. Before discontinuing a prescription medication, always check, at least by phone, with the prescribing physician, as there may be important reasons for continuing its use or there may be withdrawal reactions.

3. Are you drinking alcohol in order to feel better? Alcohol is also a downer. There is virtually no way to escape depression unless you free your brain of these negative influences. For most people, one or two drinks in the evening is not a problem, but if your mind is not totally free of alcohol during most of the day, you are having trouble with this drug.

4. Continue your daily activities. Get dressed every day, make your bed, get out of the house, go shopping, walk your dog. Plan and cook meals. Force yourself to do these things even if you don't feel like it.

5. Visit with friends. Call them on the phone, plan to go to the movies or on other outings.

6. Join a group. Get involved in a church group, a discussion group at a senior citizen club, a community college class, a self-help class, or a senior nutrition program.

7. Make plans and carry them out. Look to the future. Plant some young trees. Look forward to your grandchildren's graduation from college even if they are in kindergarten.

8. Don't move to a new setting without first visiting for a few weeks. Moving can be a sign of withdrawal, and depression often intensifies when you are in a location away from friends and acquaintances. Your troubles may move with you.

9. Take a vacation with relatives or friends. Vacations can be as simple as a few days in a nearby city or a resort just a few miles down the road. Rather than go alone, look into trips sponsored by colleges, senior centers, or church groups.

10. Do twenty to thirty minutes of physical exercise every day.

11. Make a list of self-rewards. Take care of yourself. You can reward yourself by reading at a set time, seeing a special play, or by anything big or small that you can look forward to.

12. Get a pet. Animals are wonderful, cheerful companions.

Depression feeds on depression, so break the cycle. The success of everything else in this book depends on it. Depression is not permanent, and you can hasten its disappearance. Focus on your pride, your friends, your future goals, your positive surroundings. How you respond to depression is a self-fulfilling prophecy. When you believe that things will get better, they will.

Finally, if you are unable to get out of your depression despite your best efforts, talk to your doctor. A short course of antidepressant medication and/or counseling may be needed to get you back to your old self.

PAIN

Although we have talked a lot about pain in earlier chapters, here we would like to review some basic principles and discuss the connection between pain and mood.

1. Keep active when you have pain. Get dressed in your favorite clothes. Women, put on makeup. Men, shave. Now do something. Go to work, go out shopping, go to a movie you have wanted to see. All of these activities will make you look and feel good, and will help keep your mind off the pain. If instead you stay home in your favorite old robe, stay in bed or mope around the house, you will have too much time to think about your pain and it will seem worse than it is.

2. Do your exercises. Unless you are in a "flare" and have "hot" joints, your exercises will help. Some of the pain of arthritis is due to stiff, unused muscles. Therefore, it is very important to keep your muscles in strong, supple condition. Muscle strength will also help keep your joints stable. See Chapters 10 to 13.

3. Practice relaxation exercises. Relaxed muscles and nerve endings send out fewer pain messages, thus you have less pain. See Chapter 15.

4. Don't be a martyr. Pain is individual, and it cannot be seen. Therefore, don't be afraid to tell friends and family members that you are in pain. Ask for help in carrying groceries, making beds, or mowing the lawn. Don't worry if people look at you strangely. Remember that people usually can't see your arthritis or tell that it is hurting you. A direct request for help is not being dependent; it is a direct, honest, and often necessary communication.

5. Pain is closely related to stress and depression. Thus, reducing stress and depression will also reduce pain. Sometimes people are not aware of how closely attitude and pain are related. Thus, we suggest a simple exercise. For a week, keep a Pain/Mood Diary like the one shown on page 216. Each day, put a dot somewhere between "No Pain" and "Terrible Pain" to indicate your pain for that day. Do the same for your mood. After a week, connect all the pain marks and all the mood marks. You may be surprised to see the connections between your mood and your pain.

FATIGUE

There is no question about it, arthritis can drain your energy. This is particularly true of rheumatoid arthritis and fibromyalgia, but it can be a problem in any type of arthritis.

Activities are more energy-demanding when you have arthritis, especially an inflammatory type. The body is less efficient in its use of energy reserved for everyday activities, in part because some of this energy is used in the body's attempt to heal itself.

Fatigue can have many causes such as the following:

▼ Inactivity. Muscles not used become deconditioned; that is, they become less efficient in doing what they are supposed to do. The heart, which is made of muscular tissue, can also become deconditioned. When this happens, the ability of the heart to pump blood and necessary nutrients

Pain/Mood Diary
PAIN

	SUN.	MON.	TUES.	WED.	THURS.	FRI.	SAT.
No Pain							
Terrible Pain							

MOOD

	SUN.	MON.	TUES.	WED.	THURS.	FRI.	SAT.
Feeling Great							
Feeling Awful							

and oxygen to other parts of the body is decreased. When muscles do not receive nutrients and oxygen necessary to function properly, they tire more easily than muscles in good condition—the ones that receive an adequate supply of blood, oxygen, and nutrients.

▼ Poor nutrition. Food is our basic source of energy. If the fuel we take in is not of top quality and/or in proper quantities, fatigue can result. For some people, obesity results in fatigue. Extra weight increases the amount of energy needed to perform daily activities and adds stress to joints. For others, being underweight can cause problems associated with fatigue. More about nutrition can be found in Chapter 14.

▼ Insufficient rest. For a variety of reasons, there are times when we do not get enough sleep or have poor-quality sleep.

▼ Emotions. Stress and depression can also cause significant fatigue. Most people are aware of the connection between stress and feeling tired, but fatigue is also an important symptom of depression.

If fatigue is a problem for you, your first job is to *determine the cause*. Are you eating a proper diet? Are you exercising? Are you getting enough good-quality sleep? If you answer no to any of these questions, you may be well on your way to determining one or more of the reasons for your fatigue.

The important thing to remember about your fatigue is that it may be caused by many things other than your arthritis. Therefore, in order to fight and prevent fatigue, you must address the cause(s) of your fatigue.

People often say they can't exercise because they feel fatigued. This creates a vicious cycle: People are fatigued because of a lack of exercise, yet they don't exercise because of the fatigue. Believe it or not, if this is your problem, then motivating yourself to do a little exercise next time you are fatigued may be the answer. You don't have to run a marathon. Just go outdoors and take a short walk. If this is not possible, then walk around your house. See Chapter 10 for more information on getting started on an exercise program.

If emotions are causing your fatigue, rest will not help. In fact, it may make you feel worse. Fatigue is often a sign of depression. But if the fatigue is caused by your disease, then there are several things you can do.

1. Conserve your energy (see Chapter 8).
2. Do the obvious—rest! Take a short nap once or twice a day. If this is impossible, then just relax. Try doing a relaxation exercise.
3. Fatigue, like pain and fear, cannot be seen and is not understood by most people. Therefore, tell your boss, friends, and family that fatigue is one of the problems of your arthritis and that you may have to take short rests from time to time. Most employers are more than willing to allow a little extra rest time for good employees. You, your family, your friends, and your employer should understand that there is a difference between fatigue and being lazy.

4. Take a good long look at yourself. Will you allow yourself to rest? Many of us build our self-images around the ideal of being indestructible—super-mom, macho man, or the perfect worker. If this is you, then reassess your position. Fatigue is one of the body's major early warning systems; it is telling you to take heed. Tune in to your own body and follow its directions.

CONSTIPATION

Constipation is common among people with arthritis. One reason for this is that many people with arthritis are not as physically active as they once were. Another is that a number of arthritis medications tend to be constipating.

To prevent or deal with constipation, keep these suggestions in mind:

1. **Pay attention to your body's signals.** If you feel you need to go to the bathroom, don't wait. Go. It is easier for your body to develop its own natural schedule for bowel movements when you pay attention to the warning signals.
2. **Take your time in the bathroom.**
    - ▼ Take deep breaths to relax the muscles.
    - ▼ Tuck in your belly and navel, then raise one leg toward your chest. Rest your foot on the seat if you can do so comfortably.
    - ▼ Don't strain.
    - ▼ To make sure you take your time, have something to read or a radio in your bathroom.
3. **Don't force your body onto a rigid schedule.** There is no need to have a bowel movement every day.
4. **Don't overuse laxatives.** If you don't feel pain or discomfort when you go to the bathroom, don't take laxatives to force yourself onto a different schedule.

   Laxatives can make minor problems with constipation more persistent. If you use one frequently your intestines can become dependent on it, with the result that you become constipated when you stop the laxative. If this happens, don't try to solve the problem by going back to the laxative. Instead, give your system time to adjust to functioning on its own. Help it along by following the other suggestions in this section.

   If you must use a laxative, use one based on psyllium (Metamucil, Hydrocil Instant, Fiberall, Serutan). Psyllium is a natural product that holds water and adds bulk. When using one of these products be sure to drink plenty of water or other fluid (6 to 8 glasses a day).

In general, try to avoid antacids; many can be constipating. If you must take an antacid while constipated, choose one that tends not to be constipating. Avoid milk of magnesia. (Maalox, Mylanta, and Gelusil are possible substitutes.)

5. **Manage your stress level.** Organize your work schedule to minimize your efforts and maximize your strength. For example, do all the upstairs work at one time, all downstairs work another time. Take rest periods. Also, try out the relaxation techniques discussed in Chapter 15.

6. **Eat slowly.** Mealtime should be a period of rest. When you eat, sit down, concentrate on eating, and try to enjoy your food. Don't think about problems or things you have to do. Chew slowly and thoroughly.

7. **Drink plenty of fluids.** Water adds bulk to the stool. This keeps the stool soft and makes it easier for your muscles to move it through your intestinal tract. Try to drink at least two quarts or liters of fluids each day—about eight large glasses. Plain water is good (warm or cool) but mineral water, club soda, coffee, tea, juice, milk, and soup also count.

8. **Exercise.** Physical activity will help your body eliminate waste more smoothly and easily.

9. **Eat prunes or drink prune juice.** Prunes and prune juice naturally contain a chemical substance that eases constipation. (If you are trying to lose weight, keep in mind that prune juice has more calories than most juices.)

10. **Gradually add fiber to your diet.** Our bodies cannot digest certain parts of most fruits, vegetables, and whole-grain products. The parts we cannot digest are referred to as fiber. Fiber is a natural laxative. It holds water in and adds bulk to the stool, which makes it softer and easier to expel. Fiber also helps waste pass through the lower intestine more quickly.

You can increase the amount of fiber (including insoluble fiber) in your diet by eating more fruits and vegetables and more whole-grain breads, cereals, and crackers. Both cooked and raw vegetables and fruits provide significant amounts of fiber. Whole-wheat bread is a good source of insoluble fiber, as are whole-grain cereals made from wheat. Wheat bran and bran cereal are excellent sources of insoluble fiber, but should always be eaten in small quantities with plenty of fluids. If dry cereals or wheat bran seem to irritate your system, try hot cereals instead.

Be sure to add fiber to your diet gradually over weeks or months. If you don't, you may overwhelm your digestive system, experience problems with gas, and become very uncomfortable. See Chapter 14 for more advice on fiber and healthy eating in general.

▼ ▼ ▼ ▼ ▼ ▼ ▼

18. Feelings and Communication

THE PROBLEMS of living with arthritis are not all physical ones. Many center around emotional and interpersonal issues. Just as pain and loss of function are normal symptoms of arthritis, so are the feelings of denial, fear, frustration, anger, depression, and finally acceptance. Of course, not everyone experiences all of these emotions to the same degree or on the same time schedule, just as everyone's experience with the disease is not the same. However, these feelings are important enough to merit attention.

In this chapter we will look at these feelings and discuss ways to deal with them. We will also explore some of the feelings and concerns of friends, family, and employers. Finally, we'll give you some tools for improving listening skills and communication. Not everyone with arthritis has the same set of problems. Therefore, you may not relate to all the things discussed here. As a good self-manager, take what is useful for you.

AFTER THE DIAGNOSIS

Disbelief or Denial

When someone is first diagnosed with arthritis, it often comes as a shock. "This can't be happening to me." "The doctor must be wrong." "I'm not old enough to have arthritis." These are all common thoughts. Common reactions are either to ignore the disease or, if this is impossible, to seek a "cure." The "source" of the cure may be going from doctor to doctor, trying special diets, or following the recommendations of other healers.

If you are truly concerned that you may have been misdiagnosed, get a second opinion. If you have osteoarthritis, a second opinion can come from any family doctor or internist. If you have rheumatoid or another type of arthritis, you may want to get the opinion of a rheumatologist. While a second opinion can be valuable, we must caution against going from doctor to doctor. One of the best things to do is to establish a long-term relationship with a physician whom you like and trust. Thus, as the disease changes, he or she can more easily become familiar with you and the tempo of your disease. This is probably one of the best tools any doctor can have in working with patients to manage arthritis.

Fear and Panic

Fears can surface at any time. Some people are afraid they won't be able to do the things they must or want to do. They may be afraid their family and friends won't understand. One of their greatest fears is that they will become dependent on others. Of course, there are other fears. "How can I manage a life of pain?" "My body will change, and I'll be ugly." "If I can't keep up, my partner will leave me." "I'll become a burden to my children." "I won't be able to earn a living." Probably the greatest fears of all are the fears of change and of the unknown.

First, know that your fears are normal. You are not going crazy. Next, begin to deal with your fears by seeking knowledge and by communicating. This is the time to begin learning about arthritis. However, before you start you should know your diagnosis so that as you read, you can sort out the things that apply to you. Seek out information. A good place to start is with the Arthritis Foundation or the Arthritis Society; you can find phone numbers in the back of this book. Also, go to your local library and find books on arthritis. If a book is more than five or, at the most, ten years old, the information is probably out of date and should be read with great caution. Other sources of information include your doctor, possibly your pharmacist, other health professionals such as physical and occupational therapists, and, of course, your friends.

This is also a good time to seek out others with arthritis. Join a support group such as those offered by the Arthritis Foundation. See if you can find a friend or a friend of a friend who has a similar problem. You might even ask your doctor to put you in contact with others who have some of the same problems. Meeting people with arthritis who have managed to live full and successful lives is one of the best ways to overcome fear.

Talk about your fears. In this way you may find that many of your fears are unrealistic. Recently, we did a study of the fears of children with arthritis and found that many of them were afraid of dying, which rarely occurs. In these cases all it took was a few words from a parent or the doctor to remove what was for these children a major nightmare. We have also met older people who begin to get osteoarthritis of the fingers. They are very concerned about the changes in their hands and fear that they will lose function and become help-less. Again, a few words go a long way toward alleviating fears. Osteoarthritic hands, despite deformities, usually remain completely functional.

Finally, some fears may be realistic. Arthritis may mean a change in lifestyle or relationships. However, these changes are not always negative. Many people have told us that arthritis, while not a welcomed visitor, has helped them to accomplish more in their lives and to gain greater happiness. The road from fear to accomplishment is not an easy one, but it is possible. Finding support and remaining open to new adventures will make the journey easier.

AS TIME GOES ON

Uncertainty and Frustration

In talking with many people with arthritis, we have learned that one of the most difficult tasks in living with this disease is learning to live with uncertainty. Because the disease waxes and wanes in an unpredictable manner, it is very difficult to plan anything. One day it is possible to live an almost normal "pre-arthritis" type of life, and yet the next day finds one barely able to function. "I can't plan anything." "I never know how I will be feeling." "My family is constantly postponing pleasurable activities because of my illness." "My boss gets upset because she can't count on me." "Friends don't understand when I have to cancel at the last minute." There is no way to make living with uncertainty easy. However, there are some ways of easing the uncertainty and the guilt that come from not fulfilling commitments.

Start by keeping a log or diary of your daily activities and your physical symptoms. You will learn what activities make your arthritis worse and can start rearranging your activities to do the things you need and want to do.

If there is a very important event coming up in your life, such as a wedding or a reunion, talk with your doctor first. He or she may be able to rearrange your medications for a short period of time so that you can enjoy the event without suffering the fear of uncertainty.

Plan ahead. If there is something you want to do, rest up beforehand.

Talk with your family and friends about the uncertainties. If they know your limitations, they will be more understanding.

Don't expect others to cancel plans just because you have to cancel. It is very frustrating, for example, not to be able to go to the zoo with the children or attend a party, but you can make sure that the activity goes on without you. This way friends and family won't be unduly denied pleasurable activity because of your arthritis. It will also help you avoid guilty feelings.

Anger

Not everyone with arthritis experiences anger; however, it is very common. The anger is usually aimed at an unfair world. "Why me?" "It doesn't matter what I do, nothing works." Sometimes, because of all the frustrations, the anger is expressed—rightly or wrongly—toward family and friends. "Why isn't my spouse more helpful?" "The kids shouldn't be so demanding." "Can't my friends understand that I hurt?" "My doctor doesn't believe me." Unfortunately, anger is often expressed in very unproductive ways. These include giving up, *doing* nothing. "Why bother? Nothing I do works anyway." Another way of expressing anger is *saying* nothing. Rather than expressing it in words, we may act it out in hostile actions, such as refusing to talk to a spouse or dropping a long-time friendship. Of course, the most common way of expressing anger is to shout, blow up, or be verbally hurtful. None of these expressions of anger is helpful. Rather, they often make the situation worse by alienating the very people who can be the most helpful.

First, recognize that being angry is normal. You have a lot to be angry about. This is not a fair world, and arthritis is not a fair disease. At times it may seem that nothing you do works. However, there is another way of looking at this: If you do nothing, you might get worse sooner, or you might develop more serious problems than the ones you already have. Although doing something does not always make you better, it helps to maintain the status quo. At other times it helps in slowing deterioration. For example, one thing we have learned from our studies is that for many people with arthritis, self-management does not improve their daily functioning, but it does slow the decline. That is, they still have problems of function, but instead of getting worse over time, they remain about the same. Thus, four years later, they still have the same problems, but they haven't gotten worse. A change of perspective sometimes helps.

When the anger is directed at another person, the first thing to do is determine what is making you angry. It may be that a friend is being too helpful, while for someone else the problem may be that a friend is offering no help. The second thing to do is to decide what action the other person could take that would correct the situation.

Once you have done these two things you are ready to express your anger in a way that has a chance of defusing the situation and helping you get what you need and want. One of the best ways to do this is to use "I" messages. An "I" message is one in which you express your feelings and desires rather than blame the other person. Such messages are aimed at opening up communications rather than closing them down. "I" messages are explained in detail at the end of this chapter.

Sometimes the anger and frustration of having arthritis needs to be discussed with someone besides your family and friends. This is the role of a professional counselor. Look for someone who has had experience in working with people who have a chronic illness. Psychologists, social workers, family counselors, and religious leaders such as priests, ministers, and rabbis can be very helpful. It is a wise person who seeks help rather than being hurtful to loved ones.

Depression or Sadness

Almost everyone with arthritis suffers some depression or sadness. Again, this is quite normal. After all, you have had many losses and have to make changes in your life. To learn more about depression, see Chapter 17.

Acceptance

Arthritis often means making changes in life. You may not be able to do everything that you once could. This may be due to physical disability or just a lower energy level. Unfortunately, people sometimes make the wrong choices about what they can and cannot do. One older class participant was very unhappy because he did not have the energy to join his friends for lunch. When we asked him what he did at home in the mornings he gave us a long list of chores, starting with preparing a large breakfast and followed by washing dishes, dusting, working in the garden, and assisting a friend. Clearly, he had plenty of energy, but was not using it on social activities. A woman was very unhappy because she was not able to prepare a huge traditional holiday dinner for her family. When we asked these people if they couldn't do less or ask for help, it was obvious they considered the tasks they were doing as part of their role in life. They thought that doing one's chores came before the pleasure of lunch with friends, and that a good mother fixed holiday meals.

Start by sitting down and deciding what is really important to you. When the gentleman above did this, he discovered that of all his morning activities, having a big breakfast and doing some gardening were most important. The woman decided that it was very important to make the holiday dessert, but the rest of the meal could be done by others.

Next, decide how you are going to get the other things done or what you may leave undone. The man decided that he could do dusting once a week, wash the dishes just once a day, and tell his friend that he was very sorry but that he wasn't able to help. The woman decided she could ask the different members of her family each to contribute a dish for the dinner and the older children to clean up after the meal. In fact, the family had been offering to do this for years, and the woman had refused.

Third, make a list of all the things you really want to do and then prioritize the activities. Here the important word is *want*. Next, make a list of all the things you feel you *have* to do and, again, prioritize these.

Finally, look at the two lists. If something appears on both lists, then this is an activity you probably should keep. If there are things on the "have-to" list that keep you from doing things on the "want" list, think about how you can get some of the "have-to" things done. Or maybe they can be left undone. A house doesn't have to be dusted every day.

This brings us to asking for help. One of the most important but also most difficult things anyone with arthritis can learn to do is ask for help. Because we like being independent, we tend to try to do all the things we feel must be done ourselves, and give up the things we like doing. For example, some people with arthritis will give up outings with family and friends in order to clean the house or maintain the garden, rather than asking for help in order to be able to go out.

There are several sources of help. You can ask family or friends. Many times these people would be more than happy to do some shopping or gardening. They may not have offered because they were afraid of hurting your feelings or they were not aware you needed help. Second, you can employ someone to do the tasks that have to be done but that you cannot do. Maybe a neighbor child will mow the lawn while you garden. Finally, in every community there are organizations set up to give help. Church and temple youth groups, Scouts, and service clubs all have members who want to help. Sometimes businesses let you shop by phone. Even if something seems far-fetched, investigate the possibilities. Help usually will not come without your seeking it.

FOR YOUNG ADULTS WITH ARTHRITIS

For young people, arthritis can be an especially devastating burden. It sometimes seems that all of life's promise has been taken away. This need not be so. We know many young people with arthritis, some pictured in this book, who lead full, active, work and family lives. In talking with them we learn to emphasize the 90% that can be done, rather than the 10% that must be put aside.

Young men and women with arthritis can lead full, happy married lives. It is important that the spouse understand the disease, its changeable ways, and the extra stresses that it can place on a relationship. When arthritis causes marital problems it is often for one of two reasons. The most common reason is that the spouse was not prepared for living with uncertainty. It is hard to understand how one can look the same yet on one day be fully active and on the next barely able to move. Thus, the spouse without arthritis sometimes feels put upon and may wonder if arthritis isn't just an excuse for not doing what one does not want to do.

Along these same lines, some spouses sometimes get annoyed with all the extras. As one put it, "I hate 'would you mind …?' all the time." On the other hand, other spouses have told us that they are more than happy to be of help. What is annoying and grating to one is perfectly acceptable to another.

Another problem is the spouse who is too helpful. In one case, a new mother with rheumatoid arthritis was not allowed by her husband to do anything for their baby except feed him. It is therefore no wonder that the child turned more to his father for love and support. Being too helpful can be just as devastating as not being helpful enough.

Most young women with almost any type of arthritis can conceive and bear a child. If you are thinking of becoming pregnant, it is important to discuss this with your doctor. You may need to change medications and be more carefully monitored than someone without arthritis.

Unfortunately, some young people with arthritis find themselves divorced and caring for one or more children just when they most need help. This is a sad and complex set of problems. Our suggestion is to seek and accept help. Help comes in many forms: family, friends, and neighbors, as well as professionals, including your personal physician, social workers, and psychologists.

In short, having arthritis when you are young is a challenge. However, there is no reason that, with a little thought and care, you can't lead a full and active life.

POSITIVE OUTCOMES

So far we have talked mostly about the negative aspects of arthritis. However, there are also some positive aspects. Arthritis, like other adversity, often brings families and friends closer together. Where they once took each other for granted, they now cherish their relationships and use them to the fullest.

We have even heard some people say that while no one wants arthritis, it was one of the most positive things to have happened in their lives.

For others, arthritis has become a challenge, another mountain to conquer. Using some of the techniques we outlined in Chapter 7, they set goals and worked little by little to accomplish them. Sometimes the challenges are small, such as being able to climb the steps of a daughter's home in order to share in holiday festivities. Other times the challenges are greater: arranging a trip to a foreign country to see the things one has always wanted to see. The challenges can also be personal. One elderly gentleman we know had very severe rheumatoid arthritis. His pain was such that even getting out of the house was an effort. All his life he had wanted to be a swimming instructor. With this goal in mind he had both hips replaced, underwent lengthy rehabilitation, and is now teaching swimming.

ADVICE FOR FAMILY, FRIENDS, AND EMPLOYERS

When you have arthritis, you're not the only person who has to deal with the problem. Your family, friends, colleagues, and employers, as well as many other people in your life, must also learn about and adapt to the disease. Often, however, people have misconceptions about arthritis, and may feel uncomfortable about asking you for information. Some of the most common problems and concerns are discussed below. Share this section with others so they'll know what to do to help make everybody's life easier.

Learning about Arthritis

Most people have an image of arthritis. Usually these images are either of someone badly deformed and handicapped, often bedridden, or of an older person hobbling about with a walking stick. Today, neither image is correct. Most people with arthritis are neither badly handicapped nor bedridden. They are usually able to maintain full and active lives. While it is true that many older people have arthritis, arthritis is not an old person's disease. Anyone can be affected, including infants, children, and young adults.

Learn about arthritis and rid yourself of those stereotypes. Good sources of accurate information are your physician, the Arthritis Foundation and Arthritis Society, and the references listed throughout this book.

Not Knowing What to Do

When we are faced with someone who has a problem, we often don't know what to do. Will he be insulted if we help? Should we keep asking her how she feels? Should we ignore the problem?

The correct answer is to ask. This seems very simple, but it may not be. Before giving help, ask the person, "How can I help you?" If the answer is "I don't need any help," then accept this. If the person is a friend or family member you might say, "I won't keep offering help. However, know that I am willing to help anytime. Just ask." Such a statement makes life less awkward for everyone.

Employing Someone with Arthritis

This is a big concern. The bottom line is that most people with arthritis require little or no help and can be fully employed. However, if you are considering hiring someone with arthritis, or learn that one of your employees has arthritis, ask what can be done to help if help is needed.

It has been our experience that there are two kinds of help that employees with arthritis usually need. Sometimes the workplace needs some slight modification. In our office this has meant buying special scissors, as well as a wheeled cart to move things around from place to place. Workplace modifications need not be expensive. Small things can often make a big difference and may even mean added convenience for other employees.

The second type of assistance has to do with working hours and conditions. People with arthritis often need to move frequently. They should be free to stand up and stretch. If the job requires standing, they may need to sit a few minutes every hour or so. Also, early morning is an especially difficult time for many people who have morning stiffness. If possible, these people like to come to work late and leave late. Others prefer to work only part time. Once the needs of the person are known, and working conditions negotiated, people with arthritis *can* work, and are often more reliable than those without the disease.

Dealing with Anger and Depression

It is not only the person with arthritis who suffers from anger and depression. These emotions often affect family and friends, too. "I'm so frustrated, there is nothing I can do." "I hate to see her suffer." "It's not fair, we can't do the things we used to do." "I can never count on him for anything." "Why can't I share some of the pain?" All of these things are often said, or at least thought.

First, know that your feelings are not bad or selfish. They are perfectly normal. The best way to deal with these feelings is to communicate them. This next section will give you some concrete ways in which to start. In addition, you may want to discuss your feelings with others who have a family member with arthritis. You will quickly find you are not alone. In some cases, talking with a social worker, psychologist, or marriage and family counselor may be helpful. In short, don't keep these feelings to yourself. Deal with them honestly. This will result in many benefits for you and your loved one with arthritis.

SEX

Sexuality does not cease with a diagnosis of arthritis, but the pain and burden of the disease may make the expression of our sexuality difficult. It need not be. A full, loving sex life is available to all of us.

Sexuality encompasses much more than physical intercourse; it involves our basic needs for intimacy, for affection, approval, and acceptance. It also reflects our individuality: Each of us expresses our sexuality uniquely, depending on the beliefs and values we have adopted as we grow up.

Unfortunately, these beliefs can stifle our sexual pleasure. We tend to hold on to assumptions that limit the enjoyment we will permit ourselves. "Disabled people have no desire for sex." "No one could find my body attractive." "A woman ought not to ask for sex." If we hope to appreciate and enjoy our sexuality, we must understand how these kinds of assumptions about ourselves and our loved ones inhibit us.

Here is an all-too-common example of how our beliefs can get in our way. A woman has arthritis. Her husband is afraid of causing her more pain during intercourse and, being too uncomfortable to talk about it, becomes hesitant to initiate sex. Since she is already insecure about her appearance, she mistakenly thinks that her husband no longer finds her attractive and she feels hurt and becomes a little distant. At this point, the situation serves to reinforce her husband's initial fear that he causes her pain. He may begin to feel deprived or resentful and draw away from his wife emotionally. Or he may begin to have feelings of inadequacy or helplessness about himself, with the same result: He draws away from his wife. Nobody wins; everybody loses.

Clear communication is the tool for resolving this common impasse and, for that matter, most problems concerning sex. Each partner must clearly convey his or her needs and desires to the other, or they are destined to have an unsatisfying relationship.

What do you do if arthritis pain and fatigue is a hindrance to a sexual relationship? Some ideas for coping with pain and fatigue are found earlier in this chapter. We will not address ourselves to physical positioning or technique in this book, but articles on this topic are available from your doctor or local Arthritis Foundation or Arthritis Society office. While knowledge of different love-making techniques can be valuable to someone who might otherwise be experiencing pain during intercourse, no technique or position alone will guarantee satisfaction unless there is a willingness to explore and communicate the many aspects of sexuality with one's partner.

Many of us reserve our love and trust for everyone but ourselves. We insist on seeing ourselves as unlovable, and when we do, it is not surprising that others around us come to share that view. We have to work at letting go of those "unlovable" assumptions. "Who could love my body?" "I don't deserve love." "I'm being selfish." Few of us compare very well with the magazine ideal of sexual attractiveness. If we persist in trying to live up to this ideal, we are bound to remain dissatisfied. We must instead decide that we need and deserve sexual happiness *now, just as we are.*

We have seen a bumper sticker that reads, SEX CURES ARTHRITIS. While that may not be true, sex can actually help the pain of arthritis. It seems that the excitement of sex stimulates our bodies to produce cortisone, adrenaline, and other chemicals that help to ease pain naturally. Use this information as you see fit!

A note about partners of people with arthritis. Many men and women have told us how hard it is to watch their partners suffer with arthritis. They feel helpless and sometimes guilty that they can't in some way share in their partner's distress. It is hard to live with arthritis, even if you don't have it. We suggest that you talk these problems over with other partners of people with arthritis. You can find such folks through your doctor, arthritis classes, or your local Arthritis Foundation or Arthritis Society. The important thing is to know that you are not alone and that your feelings are normal.

COMMUNICATION TIPS

"You just don't understand!" How often has this statement, expressed or unexpressed, summed up a frustrating verbal exchange? The goal in any communication between people is first that the other person understands what you are trying to say. Feeling you are not understood leads to frustration and a prolonged feeling of frustration can lead to depression, anger, and helplessness. These are not good feelings for anyone, especially people with a chronic condition like arthritis. Dealing with arthritis can be frustrating enough, without adding communication problems.

Poor communication is the biggest factor in poor relationships, whether they be between spouses, other family members or friends, coworkers, or doctors and patients. Even in casual relationships, poor communication causes frustration. How often have you been angry and frustrated as a customer, and how often is this because of poor communication?

When you have a chronic condition like arthritis, good communication becomes a necessity. Your health-care team, in particular, *must* understand you. As a self-manager, it is in your best interest to learn the skills necessary to make your communications as effective as possible.

While reading this section, keep in mind that communication is a two-way street. As uncomfortable as you may feel about expressing your feelings and asking for help, chances are that others are also feeling this way. It may be up to you to make sure the lines of communication are open.

Verbalizing Feelings: "I" Messages

Let's face it, many of us are uncomfortable expressing our feelings. Discomfort can be acute if expressing our feelings means we might seem critical of the person we're talking to.

Especially if emotions are high, attempts to express frustration can be laden with "*you*" *messages. You* can be an accusatory word, suggesting blame. Its direction is toward the other person. Its use, when expressing feelings, can cause the other person to feel as though he or she is under attack. The other person feels on the defensive, and protective barriers go up. The person trying to express feelings reacts with greater anxiety when faced with these defensive barriers and the situation escalates to anger, frustration, and bad feelings.

I, on the other hand, is not an accusatory word. It doesn't strike out or blame. When expressing your own feelings, it often helps to express them in terms of how *you* feel, not in terms of what the other person has done. Here are some examples of "I" messages:

"You" message	"Why are you always late? We never get anywhere on time."
"I" message	"I get really upset when I'm late. It's important to me to be on time."
"You" message	"There's no way you can understand how lousy I feel."
"I" message	"I'm not feeling well. I could really use a little help today."

Watch out for hidden "you" messages. These are "you" messages with "I feel …" stuck in front of them. Here's an example:

"You" message	"You always walk too fast."
HIDDEN "You" message	"I feel angry when you walk so fast."
"I" message	"I have a hard time walking fast."

The trick to "I" messages is to avoid the use of the word you, and instead report your personal feelings using the word I. Of course, like any new skill, "I" messages take practice. Start by really listening, both to yourself and to others. Take some of the "you" messages you hear and turn them into "I" messages in your head. By playing this little word game in your head, you'll be surprised at how fast they become a habit in your own expressions.

There are some cautions to note when using "I" messages. First, they are not cure-alls. Sometimes the listener has to have time to hear them. This is especially true if "you" messages and blaming have been the more usual ways of communicating. Even if at first using "I" messages seems ineffective, continue to use them and refine your skill.

One last point: "I" messages are an excellent way to express positive feelings and compliments. "I really appreciate the extra time you gave me today, doctor."

Asking for Help

Problems with communication around the subject of help are pretty common. For some reason, many people feel awkward about asking for help or in refusing help. Although this is probably a universal problem, it can come up more often for people with arthritis.

It may be emotionally difficult for some of us to ask for needed help. Maybe it's difficult for us to admit to ourselves that we are unable to do things as easily as we could in the past. When this is the case, try to avoid hedging your request: "I'm sorry to have to ask this …" "I know this is asking a lot …" "I hate to ask this, but …" Hedging tends to put the other person on the defensive: "Gosh, what's he going to ask for that's so much, anyway?" Be specific about what help you are requesting. A general request can lead to misunderstanding, and the person can react negatively to insufficient information.

General request	"I know this is the last thing you want to do, but I need help moving. Will you help me?"

Reaction	"Uh … well … I don't know. Um … can I get back to you after I check my schedule?" (Probably next year!)
Specific request	"I'm moving next week, and I'd like to move my books and kitchen stuff ahead of time. Would you mind helping me load and unload the boxes in my car Saturday morning? I think it can be done in one trip."
Reaction	"I'm busy Saturday morning, but I could give you a hand Friday night, if you'd like."

People with arthritis also sometimes deal with offers of help that are not needed nor desired. In most cases, these offers come from people who are dear to you and genuinely want to be helpful. A well-worded "I" message can refuse the help tactfully, without embarrassing the other person. "Thank you for being so thoughtful, but today I think I can handle it myself. I'd like to be able to take you up on your offer another time, though!"

Saying No

Suppose, however, you are the one being asked to help someone? Responding readily with yes or no may not be advisable. Often, we need more information before we can respond to the request.

If the request lacks enough information for us to respond, often our first feelings are negative. The example we just discussed about helping a person move is a good one. "Help me move" can mean anything from moving furniture upstairs to picking up the pizza for the hungry troops. Again, getting at the specifics will aid the communication process. It is important to understand what the *specific* request is before responding. Asking for more information or paraphrasing the request will often help clarify the request, especially if you preface your response with "Before I answer …" This should prevent the person whose request you are paraphrasing from assuming that you are going to say yes.

Once you know what the specific request is and have decided to decline, it is important to acknowledge the importance of the request to the other person. In this way, the person will see that you are rejecting the *request*, rather than the *person*. Your turn-down should not be a put-down. "You know, that's a worthwhile project you're doing, but I think it's beyond my capabilities this week." Again, specifics are the key. Try to be clear about the conditions of your turn-down. Will you always turn down this request, or is it just that today or this week or right now is a problem?

Listening

This is probably the most important communication skill. Most of us are much better at talking than we are at listening. You need to actually listen to what the other person is saying and feeling. Most of us are already preparing a response, instead of just listening. There are several levels involved in being a good listener.

1. **Listen to the words and tone of voice, and observe body language.** Sometimes it is difficult to begin a conversation if there is a problem. There may be times when the words being used don't tell you there is something bothering this person. Is the voice wavering? Does he or she appear to be struggling to find the right words? Do you notice body tension? Does he or she seem distracted? If you pick up on some of these signs, this person probably has more on his or her mind than words are expressing.

2. **Acknowledge having heard the other person.** Let the person know you heard them. This may be a simple "Uh-huh." Many times the only thing the other person wants is acknowledgment, or just someone to listen, because sometimes merely talking to a sympathetic listener is helpful.

3. **Acknowledge the content of the problem.** Let the other person know you heard both the content and emotional level of the problem. You can do this by restating the content of what you heard. For example: "You are planning a trip." Or you can respond by acknowledging the emotions: "That must be difficult," or "If that happened to me I would be sad." When you respond on an emotional level, the results are often startling. These responses tend to open the gates for more expression of feelings and thoughts. Responding to either the content or emotion can help communication along by discouraging the other person from simply repeating what has been said.

4. **Respond by seeking more information.** This is especially important if you are not completely clear about what is being said or what is wanted. There is more than one useful method for seeking and getting information.

Getting More Information

Getting more information from another person is a bit of an art, requiring special consideration. It can involve techniques that may be simple, or more subtle.

Ask for more: This is the simplest way to get more information. "Tell me more" will probably get you more, as will "I don't understand … please explain"; "I would like to know more about …"; "Would you say that another way?"; "How do you mean?"; "I'm not sure I got that"; and "Could you expand on that?"

Paraphrase: This a good tool if you want to make sure you understand what the other person meant (not just what he or she *said*, but *meant*). Paraphrasing can either help or hinder effective communication, depending on the way the paraphrase is worded, though. It is important to paraphrase in the form of a question, not a statement. For example, assume another person says:

> *"Well, I don't know. I'm really not feeling up to par. This party will be crowded, there'll probably be a shortage of chairs, and I really don't know the hosts very well, anyway."*

If we were to paraphrase this as a statement, it might look like this:

> *"Obviously, you're telling me you don't want to go to the party."*

Paraphrased as a question:

> *"Are you saying that you'd rather stay home than go to the party?"*

The response to the first paraphrase might be anger:

> *"No, I didn't say that! If you're going to be that way, I'll stay home for sure."*

Or the response might be no response, a total shutdown of the communication, out of anger or despair ("He just doesn't understand"). People don't like to be told what they meant.

On the other hand, the response to the second paraphrase might be:

> *"That's not what I meant. I'm just feeling a little nervous about meeting new people. I'd appreciate it if you'd stay near me during the party. I'd feel better about it and I might have a good time."*

As you can see, the second paraphrase promotes further communication, and you have discovered the real reason the person was expressing doubt about the party. You have gotten more information from the second paraphrase, and no new information from the first one.

Be specific: If you want specific information, you must ask specific questions. We often automatically speak in generalities. For example:

Doctor: "How have you been feeling?"

Patient: "Not so good."

The doctor doesn't have much in the way of information about the patient's condition. "Not good" isn't very useful. Here's how the doctor gets more information:

Doctor: "Are you still having those sharp pains in your back?"

Patient: "Yes. A lot."

Doctor: "How often?"

Patient: "Several times a day."

Doctor: "How long do they last?"

Patient: "A long time."

Doctor: "About how many minutes, would you say?"

… and so on.

Physicians have been trained in ways to get specific information from patients, but most of us have not been trained to ask specific questions. Simply asking for specifics often works: "Can you be more specific about …?" "Are you thinking of something particular?" If you want to know why, be specific about what you want to know. If you ask a specific question, you will be more likely to get a specific answer.

Simply asking "Why?" can unnecessarily prolong your attempt to get specific information. In addition to being a general rather than a specific word, *why* also makes a person think in terms of cause and effect, and she may respond at an entirely different level than you had in mind.

Most of us have had the experience where a three-year-old just keeps asking "Why?" over and over and over again, until the information he wants is finally obtained (or the parent runs from the room, screaming). The poor parent doesn't have the faintest idea what the child has in mind, and answers "Because …" in an increasingly specific way until the child's question is answered. Sometimes, however, the direction the answers take is entirely different than the child's question, and the child never gets the information he wanted. Rather than with *why,* begin your questions with *who, which, when,* or *where.* These words elicit a specific response.

REFERENCES

LeMaistre, JoAnne. *Beyond Rage: The Emotional Impact of Chronic Physical Illness.* Oak Park, Ill.: Alpine Guild, 1985.

Lewis, Kathleen. *Successful Living with Chronic Illness.* Wayne, N.J.: Avery, 1985.

Lorig, K. D., et al. *Living a Healthy Life with Chronic Conditions.* Palo Alto, Calif.: Bull Publishing, 1994.

Ziebell, Beth. *Wellness: An Arthritis Reality.* Dubuque: Kendall-Hunt, 1981.

▼ ▼ ▼ ▼ ▼ ▼ ▼ ▼ ▼ ▼ ▼

PART SIX

Your Medical Resources

19. Working with Your Doctor: A Joint Venture

CHOOSING A DOCTOR

THERE are many different kinds of doctors and sometimes it is difficult to know what kind to work with for what. Fortunately, most people with arthritis do not need a specialist on a regular basis. Therefore, it often is best to find a doctor who can help you with all of your health problems. For most of you, this will be either an *internist* or a *family practitioner*.

An internist has had special training in the care of adults. Internists take care of all common adult health problems, including arthritis. A family practitioner has special training in taking care of all the common health problems that occur in a family. Thus, a family practitioner may assist at the birth of a baby and also take care of grandmother's arthritis. As a general rule, the fewer doctors you have, the better coordinated your health care will be.

For people with difficult arthritis, a *rheumatologist* can be a big help. Rheumatologists are internists with additional training in arthritis and rheumatic diseases. If your arthritis is resistant to treatment, or if you have any kind of inflammatory arthritis such as psoriatic arthritis, systemic lupus, or juvenile arthritis, seek out a rheumatologist.

Most important, if you have rheumatoid arthritis, we strongly advise that you see a rheumatologist as early as possible and periodically thereafter. As we noted in Chapter 2, rheumatoid arthritis is sometimes best managed by early and continued use of the disease-modifying drugs (DMARDs). Rheumatologists are the doctors most familiar with these drugs and are most comfortable with their early use; other doctors tend to use them too little, too late.

To find a rheumatologist, look in your telephone directory or ask your doctor if he or she thinks that a referral might be of help. (Unfortunately, not

A special note of thanks to David Sobel, M.D., for his assistance with this chapter.

all communities have physicians listed by specialty.) You can also get a list of rheumatologists in your area from the nearest office of the Arthritis Foundation and Arthritis Society. An orthopedic surgeon can be of great help in particular instances; do not hesitate to ask your doctor to arrange a referral.

A word of warning: Some people spend a great deal of time and money doctor shopping. They go from doctor to doctor looking for a cure. Unfortunately, doctor shoppers lose out by not having one physician who can get to know them and build an optimal treatment plan over time. The best advice is to find a doctor you like and stick with him or her. Often, with severe arthritis, nearly all of your care should be provided by a rheumatologist.

COMMUNICATING WITH YOUR DOCTOR

For a person with arthritis, it is especially important to establish and maintain good communications with your doctor. The relationship you have with your physician must be looked on as a long-term one requiring regular work, much like a business partnership or a marriage.

Your doctor will probably know more intimate details about you than anyone except perhaps your spouse. In turn, you should feel comfortable expressing your fears, asking questions that you may think are "stupid," and negotiating a treatment plan to satisfy you both, without feeling that your doctor is putting you down or is not interested.

There are two things to keep in mind that will help to open, and keep open, the lines of communication with your doctor. How does the doctor feel? Too often we expect our doctors to act as a warmhearted computer—a gigantic brain, stuffed with knowledge about the human body, able to analyze the situation and produce a diagnosis, prognosis and treatment on demand—*and* to be a warm, caring person who makes you feel as though you're the only person he or she is interested in taking care of.

Actually, most doctors wish they were just that sort of person, but no doctor can be all things to all patients. Doctors are human, too. They get headaches, they get tired and they get sore feet. They have families who demand their time and attention, and they have to fight bureaucracies as formidable as those the rest of us face.

Most doctors entered the grueling medical training system because they wanted to make sick people well. It is frustrating for them not to be able to cure someone with a chronic condition like arthritis. They must take their satisfaction from seeing improvements rather than cures, or even in managing the maintenance of existing conditions and preventing declines. Undoubtedly, you have been frustrated, angry or depressed from time to time about your arthritis, but bear in mind that your doctor has probably felt similar emotions about his or her inability to cure you. In this, you are truly partners.

Second, in this partnership between you and your doctor, the biggest threat to a good relationship and good communication is lack of time. If you or your doctor could have a fantasy about the best thing to happen in your relationship, it would probably involve more time for you both, more time to discuss things, more time to explain things, more time to explore options. When time is short, the anxiety it produces can bring about rushed messages that are just plain misunderstood—with no time to correct them.

A doctor is usually on a tight schedule. This fact becomes painfully obvious when you have to wait in a doctor's office because of an emergency that delays your appointment. Doctors try to stay on schedule, and sometimes patients and doctors alike feel rushed as a consequence.

Taking P.A.R.T.

One way you can get the most from your visit with the doctor is to practice what we call P.A.R.T.

| Prepare | Ask | Repeat | Take action |

Prepare: Before visiting or calling your doctor, prepare your agenda. What are the reasons for your visit? What do you expect from your doctor?

Take some time to make a written list of your concerns or questions. Be realistic. If you have thirteen different problems, it isn't likely that your doctor can adequately deal with that many concerns in one visit. Identify your main concerns or problems. Writing them down also helps you remember them. Have you ever thought to yourself, after you walked out of the doctor's office, "Why didn't I ask about …" or "I forgot to mention …" Making a list beforehand helps you ensure that your main concerns get addressed.

Mention your main concerns right at the beginning of the visit. Don't wait until the end of the appointment to bring up important concerns, because there won't be enough time to deal with them properly. Give your list to the doctor. If the list is long, expect that only two or three items will be addressed on this visit, and let your doctor know which items are the most important to you. Studies show that doctors allow an average of eighteen seconds for the patient to state his or her concerns before interrupting with focused questioning. Preparing your questions in advance will help you use your eighteen seconds well.

Here's an example of bringing up your concerns at the beginning of the visit:

Doctor: "What brings you in today?"

You: "I have a lot of things I want to discuss this visit." (Looking at his or her watch and appointment schedule, the doctor immediately begins to feel anxious.) "But I know that we have a limited amount of time. The things that most concern me are my shoulder pain and the side effects from one of the medications I'm taking." (The doctor feels relieved because the concerns are focused and potentially manageable within the appointment time available.)

Try to be as open as you can in sharing your thoughts, feelings, and fears. Your physician is not a mind reader. If you are worried, try to explain why. "I am afraid that I'll become disabled from this," or "My father had similar symptoms and it got worse," and so on. The more open you are, the more likely that your doctor can help you.

Give your physician feedback. If you don't like the way you have been treated by the physician or someone else on the health-care team, let your physician know. If you were unable to follow the physician's advice or had problems with a treatment, tell your physician so adjustments can be made. Also, most physicians appreciate compliments and positive feedback, but patients are often hesitant to praise their doctors. So if you are pleased, remember to let your physician know it.

Preparing for a visit involves more than just listing your concerns. You should be prepared to describe your symptoms to the doctor concisely (when they started, how long they last, where they are located, what makes them better or worse, whether you have had similar problems before, whether you have changed your exercise or medications in a way that might contribute to the symptoms, etc.). If a treatment has been tried, you should be prepared to report the effect of the treatment. And if you have previous records or test results that might be relevant to your problems, bring them along. Plan ahead so you can be brief and use your time effectively.

Ask: Another key to effective doctor-patient communication is asking questions. Getting understandable answers and information is one of the cornerstones of self-management. You need to be prepared to ask questions about diagnosis, tests, treatments, and follow-up.

1. **Diagnosis.** Ask your doctor what's wrong, what caused the problem, what is the future outlook (or prognosis), and what can be done to prevent it in the future.

2. **Tests.** Ask your doctor if any medical tests are necessary, how they will affect your treatment, how accurate they are, and what is likely to happen if you are not tested. If you decide to have a test, find out how to prepare for the test, what it will entail, and how to get the results.

3. **Treatments.** Ask about your treatment options, including lifestyle change, medications, surgery. Inquire about the risks and benefits of treatment and the consequences of not treating.

4. **Follow-up.** Find out if and when you should call or return for a follow-up visit. What symptoms should you watch for and what should you do if they occur?

You may wish to take some notes on important points during the visit or consider bringing along someone else to act as a second listener. Another set of eyes and ears may help you recall later some of the details of the visit or instruction.

Repeat: It is extremely helpful briefly to repeat back to the doctor some of the key points from the visit and discussion. These might include diagnosis, prognosis, next steps, treatment actions, etc. This is to double-check that you understand the most important information, giving the doctor a chance quickly to correct any misunderstandings and miscommunications. If you don't understand or remember something the physician said, admit that you need to go over it again. Don't be afraid to ask what you may consider a stupid question. You might say, "I'm pretty sure you told me some of this before, but I'm still confused about it." These questions can often indicate an important concern or misunderstanding.

Take Action: When the visit is ending you need to clearly understand what to do next. When appropriate, ask your physician to write down instructions or recommend reading material for more information on a particular subject.

If for some reason you can't or won't follow the doctor's advice, let the doctor know. For example, "I didn't take the aspirin. It gives me stomach problems," or "My insurance doesn't cover that much physical therapy, so I can't afford it," or "I've tried to exercise before, but I can't seem to keep it up." If your doctor knows why you can't or won't follow advice, alternative suggestions can sometimes be made to help you overcome the barrier. If you don't share the barriers to taking actions, it's difficult for your doctor to help.

Asking for a Second Opinion

Many people find it uncomfortable to ask their doctor for a second opinion about their diagnosis or treatment. Especially if patients have a long relationship with their doctor or simply like him or her, they sometimes worry that asking for another opinion might be interpreted by the doctor as questioning his or her competence. It is a rare doctor whose feelings will be hurt by a sincere request for another opinion. If your condition is medically complicated or difficult, the doctor may have already consulted with another doctor (or more) about your case, at least on an informal basis.

Even if your arthritis is not particularly complicated, asking for a second opinion is a perfectly acceptable, and often expected, request. Doctors prefer a straightforward request; asking in the form of a nonthreatening "I" message will make this task simple: "I'm still feeling confused and uncomfortable about this treatment. I feel another opinion might help me feel more reassured. Can you suggest someone I could consult?"

In this way, you have expressed your own feelings without suggesting that the doctor is at fault. You have also confirmed your confidence in him or her by asking that he or she suggest the other doctor. (Remember, however, that you are not bound by your doctor's suggestion; you may choose anyone you wish to give you a second opinion.)

PROBLEMS

Over the years, we have heard many complaints about doctors and would like to discuss a few of these.

1. "All my doctor does is try one pill after another."
Unfortunately, there is no way your physician can know for sure what medication will work for you. You may need to try a number of medications before you find the right combination.

This trial-and-error method can be expensive. Therefore, when you start a new medication, ask how long it will be until you know whether the drug will be good for you. If you will know in a short time, request a prescription for only a week or two, with refills of the prescription permitted. In this way you can try the medication, and if it doesn't work you won't have a lot of expensive pills to throw away. Sometimes the doctor will have free sample packages available.

Don't be discouraged if you have to try several different medications. Also, don't hesitate to let your doctor know if you have problems with a medication or if it is not working. If you have a problem with a drug and do not have an appointment in the near future, contact your doctor by phone.

2. "My doctor never tells me anything about my medications."

Again, time is often a factor, or maybe you didn't ask. If you want more information about your medications, first ask your physician. If this is not satisfactory, you can ask the pharmacist. Pharmacists are an underutilized resource for drug information. Also, this book answers some of the most common questions (see Chapter 20).

3. "There is no cure; there is nothing my doctor can do anyway."

Yes and no. While it is true there is no cure for many types of arthritis, there is a great deal that can be done. Diabetes is another disease with no cure. However, insulin and appropriate medical care enable diabetics to live nearly normal lives. No diabetic would think of saying that because there was no cure, physicians can't do anything.

For people with arthritis, medical attention can do a number of things. First, just knowing what one has relieves a lot of worry; this in itself is valuable. Second, physicians may be able to prescribe treatment to make life easier. Third, with many types of arthritis, medical treatment can control the disease or keep it from progressing. Thus, while it is true that doctors often can't cure arthritis, they often can help you help yourself in living more comfortably.

4. "My doctor uses language I can't understand."

Unfortunately, doctors are so used to talking "doctor-talk" that they sometimes exclude the rest of us. They don't do this on purpose or even realize they are doing it. The situation is simple. If you don't understand something, ask. Never be afraid to speak up.

5. "My doctor ignores my ideas about self-care."

Now, this is a hard one. Often, doctors are not trained in use of alternative therapies and, like all of us, tend to downplay things they don't know about. On the other hand, physicians have a responsibility to let you know when a proposed treatment has little scientific merit or is just plain harmful. At our

Arthritis Center in Stanford, California, we get hundreds of calls a year about all kinds of treatments. We tell people what we know or don't know and try to warn them of possible harms. We, and your doctor, also feel a responsibility to prevent folks from spending large amounts of money on treatments with potential harm or no effect.

If your doctor disregards your ideas, then you have an extra responsibility to find out about the treatment. Generally, if the treatment is free or inexpensive and does not have harmful side effects, go ahead and try it if you wish. On the other hand, be very skeptical of expensive treatments (someone is making money off of you). Treatments that promise a cure, or anything with the word *miracle* attached to it, are *never* miracle cures!

6. "My doctor never listens to me."

A good relationship takes two people, people who have similar ideas and are able to communicate. If you feel your doctor is not listening to you, we suggest you discuss it. You can start by saying something like, "Dr. Jones, sometimes I feel I'm not being heard." This takes some nerve, but we can promise that it will open up the communication process.

Another way to get your doctor to listen is to be brief and to the point. You might even practice before going in. Think out exactly what you want to say; this will make it easier.

7. "I don't feel comfortable talking with my doctor."

This is a problem many of us have. We have already discussed many ways you can make communication easier. Here is one more. Whenever you want to have a serious conversation with your doctor, plan to do it while you are dressed. It is hard to feel comfortable in your underwear or an examination gown.

Sometimes the personalities of the physician and the patient just don't fit. If you have tried to open up communications and it hasn't worked, then maybe it is time to find a new doctor. Not every patient can like every doctor and vice versa. Doctors sometimes wish they had the option of changing patients. You do have this option; when necessary, don't be afraid to use it. Good patient-physician relationships are important.

A doctor's addendum: I have never seen a person with arthritis that I couldn't help. There are some individuals, however, that I have not helped. In every such case, the communication broke down. Sometimes I am short of time or short of temper. Sometimes the person doesn't listen or doesn't hear or doesn't understand. Often, a preconceived opinion is the problem. "Aspirin won't work." "My neighbor couldn't tolerate that drug." "I hardly eat a thing."

"She seems too old to exercise." "I don't think he would understand." Or a person who reports her condition as being worse never filled a prescription, stopped an exercise program after two days, decreased medication ("It was too expensive"), and never mentioned the problem. A solid half of the blame lies with the doctor. Sometimes we do not listen or we have our own preconceived ideas. No matter how hard we try we don't always get it right. But the other half of the blame lies with the patient. Tell it true and straight and we can help. This is a partnership. We don't always have to agree to get good results. But the give-and-take of direct communication is essential.

REFERENCES

Beck, Aaron. *Love Is Never Enough.* 1988.

Fries, James F. *Living Well.* Reading, Mass.: Addison-Wesley, 1994.

Fries, James F. *Arthritis: A Take Care of Yourself Health Guide.* Reading, Mass.: Addison-Wesley, 1994.

Golde, Robert A. *What You Say Is What You Get.* Hawthorn Books, Inc., New York, 1979.

McKay, Matthew, Martha Davis, and Patrick Fanning. *Messages: The Communication Skills Book.* Oakland: New Harbinger Publications, 1983.

Pantell, Robert H., James F. Fries, and Donald M. Vickery. *Taking Care of Your Child.* 4th ed. Reading, Mass.: Addison-Wesley, 1994.

Vickery, Donald M., and James F. Fries. *Take Care of Yourself.* 5th ed. Reading, Mass.: Addison-Wesley, 1993.

20. The Drug Scene:
Medications That Help Arthritis

KNOWING all about your drugs is not easy. All drugs involve complex effects on your body, and full explanations from family doctors invariably take lots of time. Unfortunately, that time is not always available to physicians. The interview with your doctor is an intensive experience, and all too frequently discussion of prescribed treatment merely serves to end it quickly. Too little time is spent on this important subject. Here, the discussions you have been having with your physician are repeated. Read the ones you need. Reread those you forgot.

ANTI-INFLAMMATORY MEDICATIONS

Inflammation

Many important arthritis medicines reduce inflammation, and you have to know a little bit about this concept. Inflammation is part of the normal healing process. The body increases blood flow and sends inflammatory cells to repair wounded tissues and to kill bacterial invaders. The inflammation causes the area to be warm, red, tender, and often swollen. To understand the potential problems of drugs that reduce inflammation, it is important to recognize first that inflammation is a normal process.

In rheumatoid arthritis the inflammation causes damage, and thus suppression of the inflammation can be helpful in treatment. In osteoarthritis there is little inflammation or the inflammation may be necessary for the healing process. So you don't always want an anti-inflammatory drug just because you have arthritis—in rheumatoid arthritis, yes; in osteoarthritis, probably no.

Aspirin and Other Nonsteroidal Anti-inflammatory Drugs (NSAIDs)

Aspirin is one of the most important drugs for arthritis. Not only is it useful itself, but it also serves as a model for understanding the benefits and problems of medical treatments for arthritis.

Aspirin is the most frequently used drug in the world and the most misunderstood. It is among the safest drugs currently used, yet we constantly hear of its dangers. It has become so familiar that people fail to take it seriously: "Take two aspirin and call me in the morning." Yet it is said to be so powerful that today the United States Food & Drug Administration would not license it if it were a new drug. The scare press reports the hazards of bleeding from the stomach or of liver damage. The same press reports the next day that aspirin may prevent heart attacks by thinning the blood. These contradictions dominate our daily encounters with aspirin.

If used properly, aspirin is a marvelous drug for many kinds of arthritis. If not used correctly, it can lead to real frustration. Read the next several paragraphs carefully; they illustrate things you need to know about aspirin specifically, but also illustrate general principles you need to know about all arthritis medications.

What You Need to Know About Anti-inflammatory Medications

1. **Understand the difference between the terms** *analgesic* **and** *anti-inflammatory*. *Analgesic* means "painkilling." *Anti-inflammatory* means that the redness and swelling are reduced. Aspirin provides minor pain relief and is helpful for headaches, sunburn, or other familiar problems. But it also can be a major anti-inflammatory agent and can actually decrease the swelling and tissue damage in rheumatoid arthritis.

   With aspirin the dosage is the difference. The painkilling effects of aspirin are best after you take only two tablets (10 grains). If you take more aspirin, you do not really get any more pain relief. You can repeat this analgesic (painkilling) dose every four hours because it tends to wear off in about that time. In contrast, the anti-inflammatory effect requires high and continuous levels of aspirin in the blood. A person must take twelve to twenty-four tablets (60 to 120 grains) each day and the process must be continued for three to four weeks to obtain the full effect. You should take high doses only with your doctor's advice.

2. **You need to know the difference between symptoms of an allergy and side effects.** When the doctor asks what drugs you are allergic to, you may mention drugs with which you have had problems in the past. Most of the time, you have had a side effect from the drug, not an allergic reaction to it.

   Allergy is relatively rare; side effects are common. Only a few people get an allergy, but everyone experiences side effects if they get enough of a drug. There are different symptoms. A skin rash, wheezing in the lungs, or a runny nose generally mean allergy. Nausea, abdominal pain, ringing in the ears, and headache usually mean side effects. An allergy is a good reason to avoid a drug in the future. If you have side effects to a drug, usually it means that you need one or another trick to get your body to tolerate the drug better, or perhaps just a little lower dose.

For most people, it is a drug's analgesic (low-dose) effects that are needed to increase comfort. For this reason there is an increasing tendency for doctors to recommend acetaminophen (Tylenol) more frequently, since this drug gives good analgesia and is much safer than the drugs disclosed in this section.

3. **You need to know about drug absorption and drug interactions.** Food delays the absorption of a medicine into your body. With some drugs the presence of food in your stomach will totally prevent the absorption of the medication. But food also protects the stomach lining and can make taking a drug more comfortable. Thus, although food may decrease the effectiveness of a medication, it also may decrease certain side effects by protecting the stomach. By and large, antacids (Maalox, Mylanta, Gelusil) act just about the same as food; they decrease absorption but protect the stomach.

Some medications are coated to protect the stomach; the coating is designed to dissolve after the tablet has passed through the stomach and into the small intestine. These coatings work for some people. On occasion, the coating never dissolves and the person derives no benefit whatsoever from the drug; it passes unaltered into the toilet. On other occasions the coating doesn't last long enough and nausea is encountered anyway.

Drugs are chemicals. Interactions between two drugs (two chemicals) are extremely common. Aspirin blocks absorption from the stomach of some of the newer anti-inflammatory agents discussed in this section. By and large, the fewer medicines you take at one time, the more predictable your response to treatment will be. Most reactions having to do with absorption or interactions with other drugs are not perfectly predictable. You may have them or you may not. The treatment for your arthritis will ultimately be unique to you. You may need to discover by trial and error some of the reactions of your own body.

4. **You need to know about drug "half-life".** When you take a drug, the blood and tissue levels of the drug rise for a time, then fall as the drug is eliminated from the body. The time until one half of the drug has been

eliminated is called the "half-life" of the drug. This is the time when the treatment effect of the drug begins to wear off and you may need another dose. For example, if you take two aspirin tablets, the maximal effect is at about one hour, and the half-life is about four hours; hence, it might be reasonable to take two tablets each four hours. Ibuprofen and tolmetin also have half-lives of about four hours. Naproxen has a longer half-life, about eight hours. Feldene and Daypro have half-lives of close to 24 hours. Intramuscular gold and Plaquenil have very long half-lives of perhaps three or four months. (All of these drugs are discussed later in this chapter.) If you have liver disease or kidney disease the half-life of the drug may be longer than usual, and a lower dose of medication (and greater caution) may be appropriate for you.

5. **You should know about dosage equivalents, generic names, and product differences.** Aspirin is subject to more hucksterism than any other drug. It is found in the drugstore in several hundred different formulations. It is "the drug doctors recommend most." Manufacturers compete to find tiny areas of difference among products which can be exploited by advertising campaigns. There are "arthritis extra-strength" aspirin, buffered aspirin, and coated aspirin. There is aspirin with extra ingredients, such as caffeine. There is aspirin in cold formulations with antihistamines or other compounds. There is aspirin that is advertised for its purity.

A standard aspirin tablet is 325 mg, and the amount of drug is accurate to government standards. You always pay more for a brand-name formulation. For arthritis, do not buy aspirin that is compounded with any drugs other than possibly an antacid (Bufferin, Ascriptin). Even then, you may find is less expensive to take Aspirin with an antacid such as Maalox rather than to buy buffered aspirin. You do not want the caffeine or the antihistamine ingredients.

Do not use a coated aspirin (Ecotrin) unless you have stomach problems with regular aspirin. Coated aspirin is more expensive and you may not get as good absorption from your stomach. All of the aspirin available commercially is pure enough for your use. If your body can tell a difference, stay with a product that seems to work for you. Otherwise, buy the cheapest USP aspirin that you can find. If it smells like vinegar when you open the bottle, it is too old and you should throw it out. If you have problems with the new child-proof caps, ask your pharmacist for a regular top.

6. **Treat aspirin and other NSAIDs with respect.** Aspirin and other NSAIDs, despite their familiarity, are not safe medications. Their side effects include nausea, headache, upset stomach, skin rash, and liver and kidney problems. These effects have been known for a long time and are generally minor.

The major side effect is the development of serious ulcers in the stomach and severe bleeding from the gastrointestinal tract. This process usually occurs silently, without any preceding symptoms. It can result in hospitalization or even death. Because these medications are so widely used, it has been estimated that in the United States serious side effects are more common with these drugs than with all other drugs put together.

This is not to say that these drugs should be feared or avoided, since in many patients, probably a majority, the good they do outweighs the risk of side effects. Yet you should always ask yourself if you need to continue long-term treatment with these or any other drug, and whether there are safer medications for you. Since these drugs are taken for symptomatic relief, if you are not obtaining such relief from one of these medications, it is reasonable to ask your doctor about discontinuing it.

Gastric ulcers from NSAID therapy are usually located around the outlet from the stomach. These ulcers form and heal periodically in most of the patients who are taking full doses of these drugs for a long time. Occasionally, an ulcer is located near one of the larger arteries to the stomach lining and severe bleeding can result. The risk of bleeding requiring hospitalization is about 1% for each year that you take these medications in full doses. The risk of death is approximately one in ten hospitalizations, or about one in one thousand patients per year of full therapy.

All patients are not at the same risk for these problems, which are more than three times as common in people over age sixty. They are twice as common in people with rheumatoid arthritis. They are higher in people who are taking corticosteroids (prednisone; see below), and more likely in people who have already had an episode of bleeding from their stomachs. They are more common in people who have had stomach problems already and had to stop using several of these drugs. They occur more commonly in women, but only because women use these drugs more. Many studies are now underway to determine more precisely which subjects are at greatest risk.

Can these problems be prevented? At this time the answer is "probably." Antacids such as Maalox seem to help prevent the upset stomach but perhaps not the bleeding episodes. Similarly, drugs like cimetidine and ranitidine, which decrease stomach acid, seem to prevent the minor symptoms more than the development of ulcers. Sucralfates may help a little, but again results do not appear definitive. Coated aspirin appears to be about 20% safer than regular aspirin.

Recently, the U.S. Food and Drug Administration has licensed a new drug called misoprostol (Cytotec), used specifically to prevent NSAID ulcers. This is a promising development and may help to deal with this serious side effect. For patients with several risk factors for stomach bleeding, a current recommendation is to consider prophylactic treatment with misoprostol. The disadvantages: Misoprostol, while preventing the development of ulcers, doesn't always help with the symptoms you may be having from the NSAID drugs. It may actually cause symptoms, particularly diarrhea, during the first few days. It has not yet been shown definitely to prevent hospitalizations and deaths, although this effect seems likely from the studies that have been reported to date. Taking any preventative medication costs money, in the case of Cytotec about US$500 per year. Our recommendation at this writing is to consider misoprostol for patients over sixty-five, for those who have had a previous bleeding episode, and for those who are already getting preventative treatment with another agent and hence would spend no more money by switching to misoprostol.

What follows is general advice. If your doctor's advice differs, then listen to your doctor. He or she is most familiar with your specific needs. The doses and precautions listed are those known at the time of this writing and are subject to changes your doctor may know about. But if you receive advice that doesn't make sense according to the principles outlined in this section, don't hesitate to ask questions or get another opinion.

Anti-inflammatory Medications Containing Aspirin
acetylsalicylic acid (aspirin)

Purpose: To relieve pain; to reduce inflammation.

Indications: Pain relief for osteoarthritis and local conditions such as bursitis. Anti-inflammatory agent for rheumatoid arthritis.

Dosage: For pain, two five-grain tablets (5 grains equals 300 to 325 mg) every four hours as needed. For anti-inflammatory action, three to four tablets, four to six times daily (with medical supervision if these doses are continued for longer than one week). The time to maximum effect is thirty minutes to one hour for pain and one to six weeks for the anti-inflammatory action.

Side effects: Common effects include nausea, vomiting, ringing in the ears, and decreased hearing. Each of these is reversible within a few hours if the drug dosage is decreased. Allergic reactions are rare but include development of nasal polyps and wheezing. Prolonged nausea or vomiting that persists after the drug is stopped for a few days suggest the possibility of a stomach ulcer caused by the irritation of the aspirin. With an overdose of aspirin, there is very rapid and heavy breathing, and there can even be unconsciousness and coma. Be sure to keep aspirin (and all medications) out of reach of all children.

Aspirin has some predictable effects that occur in just about everyone. Blood loss through the bowel occurs in almost all persons who take aspirin, because the blood clotting function is altered, the stomach is irritated, and aspirin acts as a minor blood-thinning agent. Up to 10% of those taking high doses of aspirin will have some abnormalities in the function of the liver; although these are seldom noticed by the person taking aspirin, they can be identified by blood tests. Since serious liver damage does not occur, routine blood tests to check for this complication are not required. Hospitalization for gastrointestinal hemorrhage occurs in about 1% of people taking full doses for one year.

Aspirin is not recommended when you have influenza, chicken pox, or high fevers because of the possibility of a rare complication called Reye's syndrome.

Special hints: If you note ringing in the ears or a decrease in your hearing, then decrease the dose of aspirin. Your dose is just a little bit too high for the best result.

If you notice nausea, an upset stomach, or vomiting, there are a variety of things you can do. First, try spreading out the dose with more frequent use of smaller numbers of pills. Perhaps instead of taking four tablets four times a day, you might take three tablets five or six times a day. Second, try taking the aspirin after meals or after an antacid, which will coat the stomach and provide some protection. Third, you can change brands and see if the nausea is related to the particular brand of aspirin you were using. Fourth, you can try coated aspirin (Ecotrin). These are absorbed variably, but are often effective in protecting the stomach and decreasing nausea. Although it is a nuisance, you often can get good relief from the nausea by taking a suspension of aspirin rather than the tablet. Put the aspirin in a half glass of water and swirl it until the aspirin particles are suspended in the water. Fill another glass half full of water, drink the suspended aspirin, and wash it down with the other glass of water. This is an effective and inexpensive way to avoid nausea once you get used to the taste. You can also mix the aspirin with juice or milk.

Keep track of your aspirin and always tell your doctor exactly how much you are taking. Aspirin is so familiar that sometimes we forget that we are taking a drug. Be as careful with aspirin as you would be with any drug. In particular, you may want to ask your doctor about interactions with the newer anti-inflammatory agents, with probenecid, or with blood-thinning agents, if you are taking those drugs. Pay special attention to your stomach. So many drugs cause irritation to the stomach lining that you run the risk of adding insult to injury. Two drugs that irritate the stomach lining may be more than twice as dangerous; again, the fewer medications at one time the better. Every time you talk to a doctor, be sure to describe all the drugs you are taking, not just your arthritis drugs. It is wise to keep a list of all the drugs you take and have it ready to show any doctor you visit, including your dentist.

Ecotrin
325 mg, 500 mg tablets and caplets
See acetylsalicylic acid (aspirin).

Disalcid (salsalate)
500 mg round, aqua, scored, film-coated tablet
500 mg aqua and white capsule
750 mg capsule-shaped, aqua, scored, film-coated tablet

Purpose: To relieve pain; to reduce inflammation.

Indications: For mild pain relief of osteoarthritis and in local conditions. As an anti-inflammatory agent for synovitis or attachment arthritis, as in rheumatoid arthritis and ankylosing spondylitis.

Dosage: For pain, one or two 750 mg capsule-shaped aqua tablets every twelve hours. Each 750 mg Disalcid tablet is equivalent in salicylate content to about two and a half normal-sized (300 mg) aspirin tablets. Occasionally, higher doses may be needed. For pain, the maximum effect is reached in two hours; one to six weeks are required for anti-inflammatory action to take full effect.

Side effects: Common side effects include nausea, vomiting, ringing in the ears, and decreased hearing. Each of these is reversible within a few hours if the drug dosage is decreased. Allergic reactions are rare but potentially include development of nasal polyps and wheezing. With an overdose of any salicylate that can be very heavy and rapid breathing, even leading to unconsciousness and coma.

Disalcid is being used more frequently in arthritis because it appears to be less toxic to the stomach than aspirin and the other NSAIDs, although definitive data are not yet available. Additionally, Disalcid has less effect upon the platelets, so there is less chance of minor bleeding problems. The blood salicylate level rises more slowly and lasts longer than with aspirin, therefore the drug does not have to be taken as often as aspirin.

Disalcid should be avoided during chicken pox or influenza because of the possibility of Reye's syndrome, as mentioned before.

Some physicians do not believe that the anti-inflammatory activity of Disalcid is as good as that of aspirin. Other physicians believe that the effects are identical. So it seems likely that Disalcid is less toxic than ordinary aspirin, but it is not clear that it is as effective a drug. It finds particular use in patients who have had problems with stomach upset from ordinary aspirin or who are in high-risk groups for gastrointestinal bleeding episodes.

Special hints: If you note ringing in the ears or a decrease in your hearing, decrease the dose of Disalcid; it is just a little bit too high for best results. Keep track of your Disalcid intake and always tell the doctor exactly how much you are taking.

Trilisate (choline magnesium trisalicylate)
500 mg scored, capsule-shaped pale pink tablet
750 mg scored, film-coated, capsule-shaped white tablet
1,000 mg scored, film-coated, capsule-shaped red tablet

Purpose: To relieve pain; to reduce inflammation.

Indications: For mild pain relief of cartilage degeneration and local conditions. Also an anti-inflammatory agent for synovitis and attachment arthritis.

Dosage: For pain, one or two 500 mg tablets every twelve hours. For anti-inflammatory activity, two to three tablets every twelve hours. Each 750 mg Trilisate capsule is equivalent in salicylate content to ten grains of aspirin (two usual-sized aspirin tablets). Occasionally higher doses may be needed. The maximum effect is reached in two hours for pain effects; one to six weeks are required for anti-inflammatory action to take full effect.

Side effects: Common effects include nausea, vomiting, ringing in the ears, and decreased hearing. Each of these is reversible within a few hours if the drug dosage is decreased. Allergic reactions are rare but potentially include development of nasal polyps and wheezing. With an overdose of salicylate, there can be very rapid and heavy breathing, and even unconsciousness and coma.

Trilisate has been urged as a drug of choice in arthritis because it is much less toxic to the stomach than aspirin. Additionally, there is less effect upon the platelets, so there is less chance of a bleeding problem. The blood salicylate level rises more slowly and lasts longer; hence, the drug does not have to be taken as often as aspirin.

But a controversy has arisen because some physicians do not believe that the anti-inflammatory activity of Trilisate is nearly as good as that of aspirin. Other physicians believe that the effects are identical. So, it seems clear that Trilisate is less toxic than ordinary aspirin, but it is not clear that it is as effective a drug. It finds particular use in patients who have had problems with stomach upset from ordinary aspirin. Trilisate does require prescription; it is not clear why a prescription should be required for this drug any more than for regular aspirin.

Special hints: If you note ringing in the ears or a decrease in your hearing, decrease the dose of Trilisate; it is just a little bit too high for the best results. Keep track of your Trilisate intake, and always tell the doctor exactly how much you are taking. It is possible that there may be drug interference between Trilisate and the nonsteroidal anti-inflammatory agents discussed in the following pages, so you will usually not want to take them at the same time.

Other NSAIDs

Aspirin is a nonsteroidal anti-inflammatory agent. That is, it is not a corticosteroid (like prednisone), but it is an anti-inflammatory agent because it fights inflammation. Some of the disadvantages of aspirin have been noted above. In anti-inflammatory doses, side effects such as nausea, vomiting, and ringing in the ears are common. Some people can't tolerate these side effects. Others, either ill-advised or not persistent, don't really try. Aspirin requires many tablets and regular attention to the medication schedule. So, a class of "aspirin substitutes," given the cumbersome name of nonsteroidal anti-inflammatory drugs (NSAIDs) has been developed. In common medical usage, aspirin is not included in this group. To further simplify, we use the term *anti-inflammatory drugs* in this book. In the over-the-counter market, "aspirin substitute" usually refers to acetaminophen (Tylenol), which is discussed below as a pain reliever; acetaminophen is not an anti-inflammatory drug.

There is a huge market for NSAIDs. Nearly every drug company has tried to invent one and has promoted heavily whatever has been developed. Some of these drugs have been promoted in the financial pages of the newspaper or announced in press releases before the scientific evidence was complete. Clearly, you have to be careful about what you read under such circumstances. But there is some substance to the claims. Many of these drugs are good ones. They may be better for those truly unable to tolerate aspirin. Unfortunately, they are more expensive, newer, and their long-term side effects are less well known. Present evidence suggests that some of them, such as tolectin, indomothacin, Ketoprofen, and moclofenemate, are more toxic than aspirin.

In perspective, the development of these drugs represents a substantial advance. In part, this is because of the difficult problems posed by the corticosteroids (discussed in the next section). The use of the term non-steroidal to distinguish these compounds underscores the importance of this feature. In average potency, full doses of these drugs are roughly equivalent to full-dose aspirin.

Available evidence indicates that different drugs can be best for different individuals. These drugs come from several different chemical families and are not interchangeable. You may have to try several to find the best. The major medications in this category are discussed below in alphabetical order, according to brand name. The generic name is given in parentheses.

Advil (ibuprofen)

See Motrin.

Aleve (naproxen)

See naproxen.

Ansaid (flurbiprofen)

50 mg white tablet
100 mg blue tablet

Purpose: To reduce inflammation; to slightly reduce pain.

Indications: For relief of pain in rheumatoid arthritis or osteoarthritis.

Dosage: Usually prescribed as one tablet (50 mg or 100 mg) two or three times per day. The maximum recommended dosage is 300 mg per day.

Side effects: The most frequent side effects are gastrointestinal, as with other drugs of this group. Diarrhea is a frequent problem and can be quite severe. Irritation of the stomach lining can cause nausea, heartburn, and indigestion. Occasionally, individuals note fluid retention. Allergic reactions such as rash or asthma are very rare. Hospitalization for gastrointestinal bleeding probably occurs in about one percent of those taking full doses for one year.

Special hints: For irritation of the stomach, decrease the dose or spread the tablets out throughout the day. Absorption will be slightly decreased if you take the drug after meals or after antacids, but greater comfort may result. For the diarrhea, you have to eliminate the drug and then, if it is desired, start again at a lower dose. Flurbiprofen has been found useful in rheumatoid arthritis, degenerative arthritis, and for treatment of local conditions. Perhaps because it is one of the more recent drugs to be approved, and perhaps because of the problem with diarrhea, Ansaid has not been as widely used as many of the other agents. However, like any other drug of this group, it may be preferred by certain individuals.

Clinoril (sulindac)

150 mg, 200 mg hexagon-shaped, bright yellow tablets

Purpose: To reduce inflammation; to reduce pain.

Indications: For anti-inflammatory action and pain relief.

Dosage: One 150 mg tablet twice a day. This drug also comes in a 200 mg tablet, and dosage may be increased to 200 mg twice a day if needed. Maximum recommended dose is 400 mg a day.

Side effects: Gastrointestinal side effects, with irritation of the stomach lining, are the most common, and include nausea, indigestion, and heartburn. Stomach pain has been reported in 10% of subjects, and nausea, diarrhea, constipation, headache, and rash in 3% to 9%. Ringing in the ears, fluid retention, itching, and nervousness have been reported. Allergic reactions are rare. The use of aspirin in combination with this drug is not recommended by the manufacturer, since aspirin apparently decreases absorption from the intestine. Hospitalization for gastrointestinal bleeding occurs in about 1% of those taking full doses for one year.

Special hints: Sulindac has no particular advantages or disadvantages over the other anti-inflammatory agents described in this section, except that it may cause the minor kidney side effects less frequently and therefore is sometimes used for people with heart or kidney problems.

For stomach upset, take the pills after meals; skip a dose or two if necessary. Antacids may be used for gastrointestinal problems and may sometimes help. Check with your doctor if the distress continues. Maximum therapeutic effect is achieved after about six weeks of treatment, but you should be able to see a major effect in the first week if Sulindac is going to be a really good drug for you.

Daypro (oxaprozin)

600 mg oral caplets

Purpose: To reduce inflammation and reduce pain.

Indications: For anti-inflammatory action and pain relief in osteoarthritis and rheumatoid arthritis.

Dosage: The usual daily dose in rheumatoid arthritis or severe osteoarthritis is 1,200 mg per day (two 600 mg caplets) taken once daily. For patients of lower body weight or with milder disease, an initial dosage of one 600 mg caplet per day may be appropriate.

Side effects: Daypro can cause serious side effects, including stomach ulcers and intestinal bleeding. Most common side effects are dyspepsia and abdominal pain. As with other NSAIDs, serious side effects, such as gastrointestinal bleeding, may result in hospitalization or even fatal outcomes.

Special hints: At this writing, Daypro is the newest of the nonsteroidal drugs. Its overall toxicity is probably about average. It should not be taken by pregnant or nursing women. Its principal advantage is that it needs to be taken only once a day, since it has a long half-life. The only other NSAID that needs to be taken only once a day is Feldene (piroxicam). This is a convenience feature but it does suggest caution in dosage, particularly if the patient is older or has other disease problems, since the drug might accumulate in the body. The maximum daily dose is 1,800 mg per day, but this probably should be very seldom used. Information on long-term side effects will not be available for some time.

Dolobid (diflunisal)

250 mg film-coated, capsule-shaped orange tablet
500 mg film-coated, capsule-shaped orange tablet

Purpose: To reduce inflammation and reduce pain.

Indications: For anti-inflammatory action and pain relief.

Dosage: For osteoarthritis, 500 to 700 mg daily is equal to six to ten 300 mg regular aspirin. For rheumatoid arthritis 1,000 mg daily has been shown to be as effective as twelve to fourteen 300 mg (regular) aspirin.

Side effects: This drug is generally well tolerated. Three percent to 9% of people taking this drug may have some stomach pain or diarrhea. The frequency of gastrointestinal bleeding is probably similar to that with other drugs of this class.

Special hints: Dolobid is one of the newer nonsteroidal drugs. More studies are needed to determine its usefulness when compared to that of other non-steroidal anti-inflammatory drugs. At this time, it does not seem to have any particular advantages or disadvantages.

Feldene (piroxicam)

10 mg dark-red and blue capsule
20 mg dark-red capsule

Purpose: To reduce inflammation; to reduce pain slightly.

Indications: For anti-inflammatory activity and mild pain in rheumatoid arthritis, local conditions, and sometimes cartilage degeneration (osteoarthritis).

Dosage: One 20 mg tablet once daily. Do not exceed this dosage. This is a long-acting drug, and it need be taken only once daily.

Side effects: The drug has been generally well tolerated, although gastro-intestinal symptoms including irritation of the stomach lining do still occur, as well as nausea, indigestion, and heartburn. Allergic reactions, including skin rashes and asthma, are very rare. Peptic ulceration can occur, and hospitalization for gastrointestinal bleeding is seen in 1% to 2% of those who take full doses for one year. Since Feldene is so long-lasting, concern has been expressed that it might be unusually toxic for elderly people or for people with liver or kidney problems.

Special hints: Some seven to twelve days are required before the benefits of Feldene are apparent, and full benefits may not be clear until six weeks or more. Aspirin should be avoided in general. Dosage recommendations and indications for use in children have not been established. Some patients with rheumatoid arthritis or osteoarthritis prefer Feldene, particularly because of the convenience of once-a-day dosage.

Indocin (indomethacin)

25 mg, 50 mg blue-and-white capsule
75 mg sustained-release, blue-and-white capsule
50 mg blue suppository

Purpose: To reduce inflammation; to slightly reduce pain.

Indications: For reduction of inflammation and for mild pain relief.

Dosage: One 25 mg capsule three to four times daily. For men or large women, doses totaling as high as 150 to 200 mg (six to eight capsules) may be required and tolerated each day. It is also available in 50 mg capsules and in a 75 mg sustained-release form, which needs to be taken only twice daily.

Side effects: Irritation of the stomach lining, including nausea, indigestion, and heartburn, occurs with a number of people. Allergic reactions (including skin rash and asthma) are very rare. A substantial problem, not present with other drugs of this class, is headache and a bit of a goofy feeling. Hospitalization for gastrointestinal bleeding is seen in one to two percent of those on full doses for one year.

Special hints: Many doctors find Indocin to be rather weak for treatment of rheumatoid arthritis in early stages, although it is sometimes effective in later stages. In a long-term illness, maximum effect may take six weeks or so, but you should be able to tell within one week if it is going to be a major help. This is the cheapest of the new nonsteroidal drugs, so it if works you may save money. On the other hand, it may be one of the most toxic drugs. Some studies suggest that Indocin actually *increases* the rate of cartilage destruction in osteoarthritis of the hip.

There are also some problems with absorption of Indocin from the intestine. If you take it after meals, you have less stomach irritation, but some people do not absorb the drug very well. So, for maximum effect you need to take it on an empty stomach and for maximum comfort on a full stomach. Trial and error may be necessary to establish the best regimen for you. Aspirin poses another problem. When some individuals take aspirin with Indocin, the Indocin is not absorbed from the intestine. Usually you will not want to take these two drugs together, since you will get more irritation of the stomach lining but no more therapeutic effect than if you just took the aspirin. If this drug makes you feel mentally or emotionally fuzzy for more than the first few weeks, we think that is a good reason to discuss a change in medication with your doctor.

Lodine (etodolac)

200 mg light-gray capsules with one red band or dark-gray capsules with two narrow red bands
300 mg light-gray capsules with two narrow red bands

Purpose: To reduce inflammation and reduce pain.

Indications: For anti-inflammatory action and pain relief.

Dosage: For osteoarthritis, initially 800 to 1,200 mg per day in several doses. Do not exceed 1,200 mg per day. Lodine is not currently recommended for rheumatoid arthritis.

Side effects: This drug is generally well tolerated although as with all of the nonsteroidal agents it can result in bleeding from the stomach and other gastrointestinal problems. Some studies have suggested that there are fewer ulcers with this drug than with some other NSAIDs.

Special hints: Lodine is one of the newer nonsteroidal drugs. More studies are needed to determine its usefulness when compared with other nonsteroidal anti-inflammatory drugs. It has been found less useful in rheumatoid arthritis than other drugs of this class. It may have some advantages with regard to gastrointestinal toxicity but this is not firmly established.

Meclomen (meclofenamate)

50 mg dark-yellow-and-light-yellow capsule
100 mg dark-yellow-and-offwhite capsule

Purpose: To reduce inflammation: to reduce pain.

Indications: For anti-inflammatory action in attachment arthritis, synovitis, local conditions, and occasionally degenerative cartilage changes.

Dosage: The total daily dosage is 200 to 400 mg, usually given in three or four equal doses. The drug is supplied in 50 mg and 100 mg capsules.

Side effects: This is probably the most toxic NSAID. Gastrointestinal side effects are most commonly reported and include diarrhea in approximately one quarter of patients, nausea in 11%, and other gastrointestinal problems in 10%. Over the long term, at least one third of patients have at least one episode of diarrhea. With this drug the diarrhea is more severe than with any of the other drugs of this class, and sufficiently so to require discontinuation of treatment in approximately 4% of patients. A variety of other generally minor side effects have been reported but do not appear to be at all common. Hospitalization for gastrointestinal bleeding is seen in 1% to 2% of those on full doses for one year.

Special hints: This drug was introduced in 1980, and has been used relatively little. It is probably comparable in effectiveness to the other nonsteroidal agents. It is not recommended for children, and its effects have not been studied in patients with very severe rheumatoid arthritis. It may be taken with meals or milk to control gastrointestinal complaints. Maximum effect is achieved after about six weeks of treatment, but you should be able to see a major effect in the first week if it is going to be a really good drug for you. Avoidance of aspirin and other medications while taking this drug is advisable but not essential.

Motrin (ibuprofen)

300 mg round white tablet
400 mg round red-orange tablet
600 mg oval peach tablet
800 mg capsule-shaped apricot tablet

Motrin, Advil, and Rufen are the same drug, ibuprofen, produced by different companies. The over-the-counter brands contain smaller doses of ibuprofen and are available without a prescription (see next section).

Purpose: To reduce inflammation; to reduce pain.

Indications: For anti-inflammatory action and pain relief.

Dosage: One or two 400 mg tablets three times daily. Maximum daily recommended dosage is 2,400 mg, or six tablets.

Side effects: Gastrointestinal side effects, with irritation of the stomach lining, are the most common, and include nausea, indigestion, and heartburn. Allergic reactions are rare and the drug is generally well tolerated. A very few individuals have been observed who have had *aseptic meningitis* apparently related to this drug. Here, the person experiences a headache, fever, and stiff neck, and examination of the spinal fluid shows an increase in the protein and cells. The syndrome resolves when the drug is stopped, but can come back again if the drug is given again. Occasionally, individuals may retain fluid with this medication. Hospitalization for gastrointestinal bleeding is seen in about 1% of those who take full doses of 2,400 mg per day or more for one year.

Special hints: Motrin is not consistently useful for the treatment of rheumatoid arthritis. Overall, many doctors are beginning to feel that it is one of the weaker therapeutic agents in this group. If you are not getting enough relief from it, you may wish to discuss a change in medication with your doctor. Avoidance of aspirin and other medications while taking Motrin is advisable but not essential. It is absorbed reasonably well even on a full stomach, so if you have problems with irritation of the stomach take the drug after an antacid or after a meal. Maximum effect is achieved after about six weeks of treatment, but if it is going to be a really good drug for you, you should be able to see a major effect in the first week.

Ibuprofen sold over the counter

The U.S. Food and Drug Administration has allowed the sale of ibuprofen without a prescription in a smaller, 200 mg tablet size. This historic ruling added a third minor analgesic to aspirin and acetaminophen. The decision was made after careful review of many studies indicating that ibuprofen was at least as effective as these two previously available drugs, and possibly less toxic than aspirin for relieving minor pain. Advil and Nuprin are the trade names for over-the-counter ibuprofen, and they are already heavily advertised and heavily used. Ibuprofen is now also present in many different over-the-counter medications, including Midol.

What does this mean for the patient with arthritis? Relatively little. Many arthritis patients need at least 2,400 mg of ibuprofen per day, and twelve Advil tablets a day rather than four to six Motrin is a bit of a nuisance. And it is hard to save money, since the cost per milligram is set so that it is about the same by prescription or over-the-counter. If you need anti-inflammatory doses of ibuprofen, you should be seeing your doctor every so often anyway, so do not use the availability of the product over the counter as an excuse to stay away from the doctor. Also, many health insurance plans will not pay for medication unless it is purchased by prescription. So, our recommendation remains that ibuprofen for arthritis be used on a prescription basis unless just an occasional tablet is required for pain.

Nalfon (fenoprofen)

200 mg orange-and-white capsule
300 mg orange-and-yellow capsule
600 mg capsule-shaped orange-yellow tablet

Purpose: To reduce inflammation, to reduce pain.

Indications: For anti-inflammatory activity and mild pain relief in rheumatoid arthritis, local conditions, and sometimes cartilage degeneration (osteoarthritis).

Dosage: One or two 300 mg capsules three to four times a day. The maximum recommended dosage is ten tablets daily. It is now available in 600 mg capsules, with a maximum dosage of five tablets daily.

Side effects: Irritation of the stomach lining is the most frequent side effect and includes nausea, indigestion, and heartburn. Allergic reactions including skin rash or asthma are very rare. Fluid retention is only very occasionally a problem. Hospitalization for gastrointestinal bleeding is required in approximately 1% of patients taking full doses for one year.

Special hints: For stomach irritation, reduce the dose, spread it out more throughout the day, or take the drug after meals or after antacid. Maximum effect may take six weeks or more, but you should see major benefit in the first week if the drug is going to be a great help to you. Aspirin should be avoided in general, although the evidence for its effect on the absorption of Nalfon is controversial. Nalfon is quite useful in rheumatoid arthritis and is preferred by many individuals to aspirin on the basis of better effect on the disease as well as less bothersome side effects. It has found uses in osteoarthritis, particularly of the hip.

Naprosyn (naproxen)

250 mg round light-yellow tablet
375 mg capsule-shaped peach tablet
500 mg capsule-shaped light yellow tablet

Purpose: To reduce inflammation; to reduce pain.

Indications: For anti-inflammatory action and pain relief.

Dosage: One tablet two or three times a day. Maximum recommended dosage is 1,000 mg a day.

Side effects: Gastrointestinal side effects, with irritation of the stomach lining, are the most common and include nausea, indigestion, and heartburn. Skin rash and other allergic problems are very rare. Fluid retention has been reported in a few individuals. Hospitalization for gastrointestinal bleeding is required in approximately 1% of patients taking full doses for one year.

Special hints: Naprosyn has an advantage over some drugs in this class by having a longer half-life. Thus, you do not have to take as many tablets as with the other medicines in this group. Each tablet lasts eight to twelve hours. It is one of the most popular of the drugs of this class. Generic naproxen is now available, since the original naproxen patent has expired, and is much less expensive (see next section). An enteric coated (EC) Naprosyn is now available as well and may help prevent stomach upset.

In general, if you are taking Naprosyn you should avoid aspirin, since it interferes with Naprosyn in some individuals. An exception: Small doses of aspirin (40–80 mg per day) used to thin the blood and prevent heart attacks may be used with Naprosyn. If you notice fluid retention, reduce your salt and sodium intake, and discuss a change in medication with your doctor. If you have stomach irritation, try taking the tablets on a full stomach or after antacids. Although absorption may be slightly decreased, you may be more comfortable overall.

Naproxen sold over the counter as Aleve

In late 1993 the Food and Drug Administration (FDA) approved naproxen for nonprescription use in a smaller (200 mg) tablet size, adding a fourth over-the-counter pain reliever to the previously available acetaminophen, aspirin, and ibuprofen. This drug will be more effective in some individuals, and its longer half-life means that it only needs to be taken every eight to twelve hours. You should not take more than three tablets in twenty-four hours (people over age sixty-five should not exceed two tablets) except on your doctor's recommendation. As with over-the-counter ibuprofen, we believe that most arthritis patients should be using the prescription drug under a doctor's supervision.

Nuprin (ibuprofen)

200 mg yellow tablets and caplets
See ibuprofen

Orudis, Oruvail (ketoprofen)

25 mg dark-green-and-red capsule
50 mg dark-green-and-light-green capsule
75 mg dark-green-and-white capsule

Purpose: To reduce inflammation; to reduce pain.

Indications: For anti-inflammatory action and pain relief.

Dosage: Orudis comes in 25 mg, 50 mg, and 75 mg capsules. Recommended daily dose is 150 to 300 mg, divided into three or four doses daily. Oruvail is a more recently introduced variant with a long half-life.

Side effects: Like other drugs of this group, the most frequent side effects are gastrointestinal. Irritation of the stomach lining can cause nausea, heartburn, and indigestion. Occasionally, individuals note fluid retention. Allergic reactions such as rash or asthma are very rare. Hospitalization for gastrointestinal bleeding occurs in over 1% of those taking full doses for one year.

Special hints: This is a relatively new drug of this class, but there is wide experience with it in other countries and chemically it is closely related to ibuprofen, naproxen, and fenoprofen. If you experience irritation of the stomach, decrease the dose or spread the tablets out throughout the day. Absorption will be slightly decreased if you take the drug after meals or after antacids, but greater comfort may result. Ketoprofen is useful in rheumatoid arthritis. It has found use in degenerative arthritis of the hip and for treatment of local conditions. Like other drugs of this group, ketoprofen will be the preferred drug for certain individuals.

Relafen (nabumetone)

500 mg oval film-coated tablets
750 mg oval film-coated tablets

Purpose: To reduce inflammation and reduce pain.

Indications: For anti-inflammatory action and pain relief in patients with osteoarthritis and rheumatoid arthritis.

Dosage: Therapy is usually initiated at a dose of 1,000 mg daily, then adjusted, if needed, on the basis of clinical response.

Side effects: This is a new drug, and it has been developed in part to minimize toxicity to the stomach lining. Minor stomach ulcers are less common with this drug then with most other NSAIDs and are approximately equivalent to ibuprofen when misoprostol (Cytotec) is used to help protect the stomach. On the other hand, reduction in major ulcers and in stomach bleeding have not yet been shown and experience with the drug is limited. Diarrhea is said to occur in 14% of people with this drug, heartburn in 13%, and abdominal pain in 12%. These figures are not very different from those of other NSAIDs.

Special hints: Do not exceed 2,000 mg per day. The lowest effective dose should be used if you are going to be taking the drug for a while.

Rufen (ibuprofen)

400 mg round bright pink tablet
600 mg capsule-shaped white tablet
800 mg capsule-shaped white tablet
See Motrin (ibuprofen)

Tolectin (tolmetin sodium)

200 mg round, white tablet
400 mg orange capsule

Purpose: To reduce inflammation; to reduce pain.

Indications: For anti-inflammatory action and pain relief.

Dosage: Two 200 mg tablets three or four times daily. Maximum recommended dosage is 2,000 mg, or ten tablets daily. Larger tablet sizes may soon be available.

Side effects: Like other drugs of this group, the most frequent side effects are gastrointestinal. Irritation of the stomach lining can cause nausea, heartburn, and indigestion. Occasionally, individuals note fluid retention. Allergic reactions such as rash or asthma are very rare. Hospitalization for gastrointestinal bleeding occurs in about 1% of those taking full doses for one year.

Special hints: For irritation of the stomach, decrease the dose or spread the tablets out throughout the day. Absorption will be slightly decreased if you take the drug after meals or after antacids, but greater comfort may result. Aspirin and other drugs of this class may potentially interfere with absorption and the best rule is to take just one drug at a time. Tolectin is useful in rheumatoid arthritis. It has found use in degenerative arthritis of the hip and for treatment of local conditions. Certain individuals will prefer Tolectin to all other drugs of the group.

Toradol (ketorolac)

10 mg tablets

Purpose: To reduce inflammation and reduce pain.

Indications: For short-term relief of pain, as in a postsurgical period. Toradol is not recommended for long-term use. Generally it is not indicated for arthritis, except over periods of a week or less.

Dosage: One mg tablets every four to six hours for a limited duration only.

Side effects: Toradol, like other drugs of its class, is not free of side effects. Side effects of these drugs can cause discomfort and, rarely, there are more serious side effects, such as gastrointestinal bleeding, which may result in hospitalization and even fatal outcomes.

Special hints: This is a new drug and should be used with great caution, since all of its side effects may not be known.

Voltaren, Cataflam (diclofenac)

25 mg round, film-coated yellow tablet
50 mg round, film-coated light-brown tablet
75 mg round, film-coated white tablet

Purpose: To reduce inflammation; to reduce pain.

Indications: For anti-inflammatory action and pain relief.

Dosage: Usually one tablet (25 mg, 50 mg, or 75 mg) given two or three times a day. The maximum recommended dosage is 200 mg per day.

Side effects: The most frequent side effects are gastrointestinal, as with other drugs of this group; irritation of the stomach lining can cause nausea, heartburn, and indigestion. Occasionally, individuals may note fluid retention. Allergic reactions such as rash or asthma are very rare. Hospitalization for gastrointestinal bleeding probably occurs in about 1% of those taking full doses for one year.

Special hints: Voltaren, one of the more recently released nonsteroidal medications in the United States, has had extensive use internationally. In fact, it is the most frequently used nonsteroidal medication worldwide. The FDA was slow to review it, in part because of fear of its leading to more frequent liver problems. This does not appear to be the case, but periodic blood tests for liver toxicity are recommended by some.

Voltaren comes with an "enteric coating" designed to improve stomach tolerance; this is probably not effective. In case of irritation of the stomach, decrease the dose or spread the tablets out throughout the day. Absorption will be slightly decreased if you take the drug after meals or after antacids, but greater comfort may result.

Voltaren is useful in rheumatoid arthritis, degenerative arthritis, and treatment of local conditions. Certain individuals will prefer Voltaren over other drugs of this group. Cataflam is a derivative drug recently released; its uses are in short-term pain relief and not arthritis treatment.

Soon-to-be-Released Nonsteroidal Medications

A number of new, nonsteroidal anti-inflammatory drugs (NSAIDs), relatively similar to those just discussed, are in the process of review by the Food and Drug Administration of the United States. Many of these drugs are currently being used in other countries and appear to have a role in the treatment of arthritis. The review process by the FDA now takes approximately four to five years, and it is not possible to predict whether or not a new agent will be released or after what period. Judging on the basis of current knowledge, none of these new drugs will be dramatically different from drugs already available, so not too much is being lost by these delays. Also, a new drug is less well understood in terms of toxicity and benefits than a drug that has already been widely used. On the other hand, individual patients often do better with one or another nonsteroidal drug, so a wide choice of drugs is helpful for finding the drug that causes you the least toxicity and gives you the most benefit.

Some of these drugs have been formulated to have less gastrointestinal toxicity than their predecessors, and they may actually be safer agents. Often, on the other hand, the agents that cause the fewest side effects turn out to be the least powerful drugs for the management of arthritis.

In general, when considering one of the new agents, rely on your doctor's advice. Acetaminophen (Tylenol) is the safest pain reliever. If you have been having a lot of trouble with stomach upset from drugs, then it might be a good idea to try one of the agents that causes less gastrointestinal difficulty such as Disalcid, Trilisate, Relafen, or ibuprofen. If you have not been getting the desired effect from the drugs of one chemical class, sometimes it is useful to try the drugs of a different class. It is possible that some new drugs will be better for rheumatoid arthritis and others better for osteoarthritis or other forms of arthritis. But treat each of these drugs with respect and consider that it is always possible for a drug, particularly a new drug, to be responsible for a new symptom problem that develops while you are taking the medication.

CORTICOSTEROIDS

About 1950, a widely heralded miracle occurred: the introduction of cortisone for the treatment of rheumatoid arthritis. The Nobel Prize for Medicine was awarded to the doctors who developed this drug. People with rheumatoid arthritis and other forms of synovitis suddenly noted that the swelling and pain in their joints decreased and that the overall toxicity of the disease disappeared. They felt fine.

The initial enthusiasm for cortisone in arthritis was tremendous. But over the following years a number of major cautions began to be voiced. Slowly, the cumulative side effects of the cortisonelike drugs began to be recognized. For many individuals, the side effects were clearly greater than any benefits obtained. Cortisone became the model of a drug that provides early benefits but late penalties. Now, with a quarter of a century of experience with corticosteroids, our perspective is more complete. They represent a major treatment for arthritis, but their use is appropriate in only a relatively few cases and then only with attention to potential complications.

Steroids are natural hormones manufactured by the adrenal glands. When used medically, they are given in doses somewhat higher than the amounts the body generally makes. In these doses they suppress the function of your own adrenal glands and lead to a kind of drug dependency as the gland slowly shrinks. After many months of steroid use, the drug must be withdrawn slowly to allow your own adrenal gland to return to full function; otherwise an "adrenal crisis" can occur in which you just don't have enough hormone. Steroids must be taken exactly as directed, and a physician's close advice is always required.

Steroids used in treating arthritis are very different from the sex steroids, or androgens, taken by athletes, which have no role in treating arthritis and, indeed, shouldn't be used by athletes either.

Let's discuss the side effects. They can be divided into categories depending upon the length of time you have been taking the steroid and the dose prescribed. Side effects result from a combination of how high the dose is and how long you have been taking it. If you have been taking steroids for less than one week, side effects are quite rare, even if the dose has been high.

If you have been taking high doses for one week to one month, you are at risk for development of ulcers, mental changes including psychosis or depression, infection with bacterial germs, or acne over the skin. The side effects of steroid treatment become most apparent after one month to one year of medium to high dosage. The individual becomes fat in the central parts of the body, with a buffalo hump on the lower neck and wasting of the muscles in the arms and legs. Hair growth increases over the face, skin bruises appear, and stretch marks develop over the abdomen. After years of steroid treatment (even with low doses) there is loss of calcium, resulting in fragile bones. Fractures can occur with only slight injury, particularly in the spine. Cataracts slowly develop and the skin becomes thin and translucent. Some physicians believe that hardening of the arteries occurs more rapidly and that there may be complications of inflammation of the arteries.

Many of these side effects will occur in everyone who takes sufficient doses of cortisone or its relatives for a sufficient period of time. The art of managing arthritis with corticosteroids involves knowing how to minimize these side effects. The physician will work with you to keep the dose as low as possible at all times. If possible, you may be instructed to take the drug only once daily rather than several times daily, since there are fewer side effects when it is taken this way. If you are able to take the drug only every other day, this is even better, for the side effects are then quite minimal. Unfortunately, many people find that the dosage schedules that cause the fewest side effects also give them the least relief.

Steroids are always to be used with great respect and caution. The tendency is slightly increasing for experienced doctors to use low-dose corticosteroid treatment in a few patients with rheumatoid arthritis, demonstrating that the proper indications for use of these drugs are still somewhat controversial. High-dose cortisone treatment for uncomplicated rheumatoid arthritis has long been considered bad medical practice in the United States; it remains the essence of some quack treatments of arthritis, such as those available in Mexican border towns. Corticosteroids are harmful in infectious arthritis and should not be given by mouth in local conditions or in osteoarthritis.

There are two ways to give corticosteroids: by mouth or by injection into the painful area. Prednisone is the steroid usually given by mouth and is the reference steroid discussed here. There are perhaps ten different steroid drugs now available. Prednisone, methylprednisolone, Decodrone, and Aristocort are among the most commonly used. The fluorinated steroids, such as triamcinolone, cause greater problems with muscle wasting than does prednisone. The steroids sold by brand name are about twenty times as expensive as prednisone and do not have any major advantages. Hence, there is little reason to use any of these other compounds. Use prednisone.

Prednisone

Doses of 1 mg to 50 mg available

Purpose: To reduce inflammation: to suppress immunological responses.

Indications: For suppression of serious systemic manifestations of connective tissue disease, such as kidney involvement. In selected cases, for use in low dose suppressing the inflammation of rheumatoid arthritis.

Dosage: The normal body makes the equivalent of about 5 to 7.5 mg of prednisone each day. "Low-dose" prednisone treatment is from 5 to 10 mg. A "moderate dose" ranges from 15 to 30 mg per day and a "high dose" from 40 to 60 mg per day, or even higher. The drug is often most effective when given in several doses throughout the day, but side effects are least when the same total daily dose is given as infrequently as possible.

Side effects: Prednisone causes all of the side effects of the corticosteroids described above. Allergy is extremely rare. Side effects are related to dose and to duration of treatment. The side effects are major and include fatal complications. Psychological dependency often occurs and complicates efforts to get off the drug once you have begun.

Special hints: Discuss the need for prednisone very carefully with your doctor before beginning. The decision to start steroid treatment for a chronic disease is a major one and you want to be sure that the drug is essential. You may want a second opinion if the explanation does not completely satisfy you. When you take prednisone, follow your doctor's instructions very closely. With some drugs it does not make much difference if you start and stop them on your own, but prednisone must be taken extremely regularly and exactly as prescribed. You will want to help your doctor decrease your dose of prednisone whenever possible, even if this does cause some increase in your symptoms.

A strange thing can happen when you reduce the dose of prednisone; a syndrome called *steroid fibrositis* can cause increased stiffness and pain for a week to ten days after each dose reduction. Sometimes this is wrongly interpreted as a return of the arthritis and the reduction in dosage is unnecessarily stopped. If you are going to take prednisone for a long time, ask your doctor about taking some vitamin D along with it. There is some evidence that the loss of bone, the most critical long-term side effect, can be reduced if you take vitamin D (usually prescribed as 50,000 units once or twice a month) together with adequate calcium.

If you are having some side effects, ask your doctor about once-a-day or every-other-day use of the prednisone. Watch your salt and sodium intake and keep it low, since there is already a tendency to retain fluid with prednisone. Watch your diet as well, since you will be fighting a tendency to put on fat. If you stay active and limit the calories you take in, you can minimize many of the ugly side effects of the steroid medication and can improve the strength of the bones and the muscles. If you are taking a corticosteroid other than prednisone by mouth, ask your physician if it is all right to switch to the equivalent dose of prednisone.

Steroid Injections

Depo-medrol, other brands

Purpose: To reduce inflammation in a local area.

Indications: Noninfectious inflammation and pain in a particular region of the body. Or, a widespread arthritis with one or two areas causing most of the problem.

Dosage: Dosage varies depending on the preparation and purpose. The frequency of injection is more important. Usually injections should be no more than every six weeks. Many physicians set a limit of three injections in a single area.

Side effects: Steroid injections resemble a very short course of prednisone by mouth and therefore have few side effects. They result in a high concentration of the steroid in the area that is inflamed and can have quite a pronounced effect in reducing this inflammation. If a single area is injected many times, the injection appears to cause damage in that area. This has resulted in serious problems in frequently injected areas, such as the elbows of baseball pitchers. Some studies suggest that as few as ten injections in the same place can cause increased bone destruction; hence, most doctors stop injecting well before this time.

Special hints: If one area of your body is giving you a lot of trouble, an injection frequently makes sense. The response to the first injection will tell you quite accurately how much sense it makes. If you get excellent relief that lasts for many months, reinjection is indicated if the problem returns. The steroid injections contain a "long-acting" steroid, but it is in the body for only a few days. The effects may last much longer than this, however, since a cycle of inflammation and injury may be broken by the injection. If you get relief for only a few days, then injection is not going to be a very useful treatment for you. If you get no relief at all or an increase in pain, this is an obvious sign that other kinds of treatment should be sought. If you can find a "trigger point" on your body where pressure reproduces your major pain, then injection of this trigger point is frequently beneficial. Occasionally, persons with osteoarthritis get benefit from injections, but injections are usually not helpful unless there is inflammation in the area.

DISEASE-MODIFYING ANTIRHEUMATIC DRUGS (DMARDs)

The anti-inflammatory drugs discussed earlier are symptomatic medications only. They don't do anything basic to control arthritis. In rheumatoid arthritis and other forms of synovitis, however, there is a much more important class of drugs. Collectively, these drugs are usually called disease-modifying antirheumatic drugs or DMARDs. They have also been called slow-acting antirheumatic drugs (SAARDs) or, inappropriately, remission-inducing drugs (RIDs). While they rarely induce true remission, they are much more effective anti-inflammatory agents than the NSAIDs and in a number of cases have been shown to slow the process of joint destruction in rheumatoid arthritis.

A revolution in thinking about rheumatoid arthritis treatment is occurring. It used to be thought the DMARDs should be reserved for late use in patients with exceptionally severe disease that could not be controlled with lesser agents. Now it is increasingly recognized that these drugs should be started early in the course, and should be regarded as the backbone of treatment for rheumatoid arthritis. In general, patients with significant rheumatoid arthritis should be on one or another of these agents throughout the entire course of their disease. If you suspect rheumatoid arthritis, you should see a rheumatologist familiar with the use of DMARDs *as early as possible.*

This shift from considering DMARDs as powerful drugs to be kept in reserve to considering them as front-line treatment came about because of a recognition of the serious complications of rheumatoid arthritis, the substantial side effects related to gastrointestinal bleeding from the NSAIDs, a reassuring safety profile for these stronger drugs, and the availability of a larger number of drugs of this class. Usually the good effects from these agents only last a year or so, and so a strategy of sequentially using them one after another (or even in combination) is required.

There are now eight of these agents available, and more are under development. These are intramuscular gold, oral gold, D-penicillamine, hydroxychloroquine, sulfasalazine, methotrexate, azathioprine, and cyclosporine. Methotrexate has become the most frequently used of these agents.

Gold Salts and Penicillamine

These are major-league drugs, although no one knows exactly why they are so effective in so many individuals. They provide dramatic benefits to over two-thirds of persons with severe rheumatoid arthritis. Each has major side effects that require stopping treatment for at least one quarter of the users and that may in rare cases be fatal. Gold salts and penicillamine are two very different kinds of drugs, but there are striking similarities in the type and magnitude of good effects and in the type of side effects. Neither appears to be of use in any category other than rheumatoid arthritis, but the scientific proof of their effectiveness in rheumatoid arthritis is impressive.

These agents can result in remission of the arthritis. In perhaps one quarter of users the disease will actually be so well controlled that neither doctor nor patient can find any evidence of it. Usually these drugs have to be continued in order to maintain the remission, but, to reduce inflammation, the effects can be more dramatic than with any other agent, except possibly methotrexate or azathioprine. Individuals who use these drugs must accept certain significant hazards, but there is a good chance of very major benefit. In rheumatoid arthritis, these drugs have also been shown to retard the process of joint destruction.

If you are not able to tolerate one of these drugs, you may be able to tolerate the other. If you don't get a good response from one, you may from the other. After failure with one drug, the chances decrease a little, but success with the second drug is still common.

Which should be used first? No one knows. In England, penicillamine is usually used first. In the United States, it is gold. Gold requires a visit to the doctor every week for a while. With costs of blood tests, the total dollar cost of the initial course of injectable gold may be US$1,200 or more. Penicillamine can be taken by mouth, and while the drug itself is expensive, the total cost may be less. In terms of effectiveness and in risk, you can consider these two drugs about the same.

Myochrisine, Solganol (gold salts)

Purpose: To reduce inflammation and retard disease progression.

Indications: Rheumatoid arthritis and some other forms of synovitis.

Dosage: 50 mg per week by intramuscular injection for twenty weeks, then one to two injections per month thereafter. Many doctors use smaller doses for the first two injections to test for allergic reactions to the injections. Sometimes doctors will give more or less than this standard dosage depending upon your body size and response to treatment. "Maintenance" gold treatment refers to injections after the first twenty weeks (which result in about 1,000 mg of total gold). The dosage and duration of maintenance therapy varies quite a bit; with good responses, the gold maintenance may be continued for many years, with injections given every two to four weeks.

Side effects: The gold salts accumulate very slowly in the tissues of the joints and in other parts of the body. Hence, side effects usually occur only after a considerable amount of gold has been received, although allergic reactions can occur even with the initial injection. The major side effects have to do with the skin, the kidneys, and the blood cells. The skin may develop a rash, usually occurring after ten or more injections, with big red spots or blotches, often itchy. If the rash remains a minor problem, the drug may be cautiously continued, but occasionally a very serious rash occurs following gold injections.

The kidney can be damaged so that protein leaks out of the body through the urine. This is called *nephrosis* or the *nephrotic syndrome* if it is severe. When it is recognized and the drug is stopped, the nephrosis usually goes away, but cases have been reported in which it did not reverse. The blood cell problems are the most dangerous. They can affect either the white blood cells or the platelets, those blood cells that control the clotting of the blood. In each case, the gold causes the bone marrow to stop making the particular blood cell. If the white cells are not made, the body becomes susceptible to serious infections that can be fatal. If the platelets are not made, the body is subject to serious bleeding episodes that can be fatal. These problems almost always reverse when the drug is stopped, but reversal may take a number of weeks, during which time the person is at risk for a major medical problem.

There are other side effects, such as ulcers in the mouth, a mild toxic effect on the liver, or nausea, but they usually are not as troublesome as the side effects just described. Overall, about one quarter of users have to stop their course of treatment because of the side effects. One or 2% of users experience a significant side effect; the other users don't really notice very much of a problem, even though a serious side effect may be about to occur. Less than one in a thousand times there may be a fatal side effect. With careful monitoring, the drug is reasonably safe and its benefits justify its use, since over 70% of those treated with gold show moderate or marked improvement. However, you must maintain your respect for this treatment and keep up regular blood tests to detect early side effects. One final note: Most side effects occur during the initial period of twenty injections. Serious side effects during the maintenance period are less common.

Special hints: You must learn to be patient with gold treatment. The gold accumulates slowly in the body and good responses are almost never seen in the first ten weeks of treatment. Improvement begins slowly after that and major improvement is usually evident by the end of 1,000 mg, or twenty weeks. Similarly, if the drug is stopped, it requires many months before the effect is totally lost. In one famous study, the gold group was still doing better than the control group two years after the drug had been stopped, although most of the effect of the drug had been lost by that time. After a side effect has been dealt with or has subsided, many doctors will suggest that the drug be tried again. Often, this can be worthwhile if the approach is very cautious, since the drug is frequently tolerated the second time around. At our Arthritis Center we do not try gold salts again if there has been a problem with the blood, but we will use it again cautiously after mild skin reactions or mild amounts of protein loss through the urine.

To minimize the chance of serious side effects, most doctors recommend checking the urine for protein leakage and the white cells and the platelets, and asking the patient about skin rash before every injection. This is good practice. Unfortunately, the combination of twenty doctor visits, twenty injections, twenty urinalyses, twenty blood counts, and so forth, makes the cost of initiating gold treatment approximately $1,200 when pursued in this manner. There are some ways to decrease this cost while preserving safety. You can ask your doctor to prescribe some test kits so that you can test your urine for protein at home. This is a very easy technique. You can ask if it is possible to have just a platelet smear and a white count rather than a complete blood count each time. You can inquire whether it is possible to have the nurse give an injection after checking the blood count without actually having a doctor visit every week. And some people have successfully been giving themselves their own shots at home with the help of a family member, although this is not acceptable to many. By using such techniques, you can save half to three quarters of the cost of a course of gold treatment.

Ridaura (auranofin)

3 mg brown-and-white capsule with tapered ends

Purpose: To reduce inflammation in rheumatoid arthritis and retard disease progression. (This drug is "oral gold.")

Indications: For anti-inflammatory activity in rheumatoid arthritis.

Dosage: Average dosage is 6 mg daily. The drug is slowly absorbed and distributed through the body, and weeks to months may be required before full therapeutic effect is achieved.

Side effects: The most common side effect is dose-related diarrhea, which occurs at some time in approximately one third of treated patients and requires discontinuation in 10% to 20% of patients. Skin rash has occurred in 4%, mild kidney problems in 1%, and problems with the platelets in .5% of patients.

Special hints: Ridaura, useful in rheumatoid arthritis, is an important drug for some patients. It is not believed to be effective in osteoarthritis, gout, or minor rheumatic conditions. It may or may not have an eventual role in psoriatic arthritis, ankylosing spondylitis, and the arthritis of children. If diarrhea is encountered, the dose should be reduced. As with intramuscular gold injections, patients should be monitored periodically for blood complications, skin rash, and protein loss in the urine. Follow your doctor's advice for the particular tests required and the frequencies with which they are needed. Ridaura is most useful in the first year or so of rheumatoid arthritis.

Penicillamine (cuprimine)

125 mg gray-and-yellow capsule
250 mg yellow capsule

Purpose: To reduce inflammation and retard disease progression.

Indications: Rheumatoid arthritis and some other forms of synovitis.

Dosage: Usually 250 mg (one tablet or two 125 mg tablets) per day for one month, then two tablets (500 mg) a day for one month, then three tablets (750 mg) per day for one month, and finally four tablets (1,000 mg) per day. Dosage is usually not increased rapidly, and may be increased even more slowly than this. After remission, the drug can be continued indefinitely, usually at a reduced dosage. And if a good result is obtained earlier, you can stop with the lower dose.

Side effects: These closely parallel those noted above for gold injections. The major side effects are skin rash, protein leakage through the urine, or a decrease in production of the blood cells. Additionally, individuals may have nausea, and some notice a metallic taste in their mouth or a decreased sense of taste.

Penicillamine weakens the connective tissue so that the healing of a cut is delayed, and a scar may not have the same strength it would have without the penicillamine. So, stitches following a cut should be left in for a longer period of time, and wound healing should be expected to be delayed. Surgery under these circumstances may be more difficult.

Special hints: Penicillamine takes a number of months to reach its full therapeutic effect and the effect persists for a long time after you stop taking the drug. Responses usually take from three to six months but can be as late as nine months after the drug is begun. Because of the risk of side effects, doctors have now adopted the "go low, go slow" approach given in the dosage schedule above. When full doses were begun earlier, the frequency of side effects was higher. Even now, only about three quarters of individuals will complete the treatment and the remainder will have some side effects, approximately the same as those listed for gold salts. The drug may be tried again after a side effect if the side effect has been mild. We do not try the drug again if there has been a problem with the blood counts, but may cautiously try it if there has been a minor problem with protein in the urine, a minor skin rash, or minor nausea.

Monitoring for side effects has to be carefully performed. Usually a blood count or smear, a urinalysis to test for protein leakage, and questioning of the person about side effects are required every two weeks or even more frequently. It should be noted that with both penicillamine and gold, careful monitoring improves your chances of not having a serious side effect, but does not eliminate them. These drugs contain an intrinsic hazard that no physician can eliminate. As with gold treatment, you can negotiate to have some of the drug monitoring done by a local laboratory and review the results yourself, check your own urine for protein, and so forth, if you desire. Most doctors who use these drugs a good deal have evolved some method of minimizing the cost of the monitoring. Again, after the first six months, side effects are relatively rare but still do occur. Some individuals will have an excellent response to the penicillamine even though they never get up to the full dosage of 1,000 mg per day.

Plaquenil (hydroxychloroquine)

200 mg scored, round white tablet

Purpose: To reduce inflammation and to retard disease progression in rheumatoid arthritis; to reduce disease activity in systemic lupus erythematosus.

Indications: Rheumatoid arthritis and systemic lupus erythematosus

Dosage: One to two tablets (200 to 400 mg) per day.

Side effects: This is the best tolerated of all drugs used for rheumatoid arthritis, and side effects are unusual. With a very few people, gastric upset or muscular weakness may result. Consideration needs to be given to the possibility of eye toxicity, which is an occasional complication of antimalarial drugs. This is a rare complication and appears to be always reversible if the possibility is regularly monitored by periodic eye examinations after the first year of treatment. The eye examination will detect any problems well before you notice any change in vision.

Special hints: Plaquenil takes six weeks to begin to show an effect, and full effect can take up to twelve weeks, so plan on at least a twelve-month trial. The eye complications appear to be much less common with Plaquenil than with chloroquine, the antimalarial drug that was first developed. They seldom if ever are seen with less than one year of treatment at recommended dosage. Bright sunlight seems to increase the frequency of eye damage, so we recommend using sunglasses and wide-brimmed hats for sun protection. We recommend eye examinations after one year of continuous treatment and at six- to twelve-month intervals thereafter. This should give ample warning of any problems. Do not exceed two tablets daily. Since the drug is so well tolerated, both tablets may be taken together in the morning. The good effects of this drug are long-lasting, and continue for weeks or months after the drug is stopped. Overall, this is the safest drug available for treatment of rheumatoid arthritis and lupus; it should be used with respect but not fear.

Azulfidine (sulphasalazine)

Azulfidine EN-tabs: 500 mg film-coated orange tablets

Purpose: To reduce inflammation and to retard disease progression in rheumatoid arthritis.

Indications: Rheumatoid arthritis and some other forms of synovitis.

Dosage: Three or four 500 mg tablets daily, taken spread out as two or three doses over the day. Dosage may be increased to as many as six 500 mg tablets, usually taken as two tablets three times daily.

Side effects: This is a sulfa drug, and should not be taken by people with an allergy to sulfa which is present in many antibiotics such as Septra or Gantrisin. Allergy is unusual, and may take the form of a rash, wheezing, itching, fever, or jaundice. Azulfidine may cause gastric distress or other side effects in some patients. Blood tests should be done every so often to detect any (rare) effects on the blood cells or platelets. Most people, probably four out of five, experience no trouble whatsoever.

Special hints: Azulfidine is used in patients with inflammatory problems with the bowels, where it reduces the inflammation, at least in part because of an antibiotic effect on the bacteria that live in the bowel. Recently, British scientists have found that it has a major effect on rheumatoid arthritis, and this has been confirmed by investigators in the United States. No one knows how it works, but it is very effective in some patients. It takes a month or more before the effects begin to be noticed, and full effects may take three or more months. Usually if you are not going to tolerate the drug, you will know in a week or so.

IMMUNOSUPPRESSANT DRUGS

Immunosuppressant drugs are very important agents for the management of rheumatoid arthritis. They are prescribed in certain cases of rheumatoid arthritis because they can reduce the number of inflammatory cells present around the joint.

The immune response helps the body recognize and fight foreign particles and viruses. When it goes wrong, it can cause allergy or autoimmune disease. In this case, antibodies from the immune system attack the body's own tissues, causing disease. Immunosuppressant drugs can tone down this reaction.

Some of these drugs work by *cytotoxic* action. They kill rapidly dividing cells much like an X-ray beam. Since in some diseases the most rapidly dividing cells are the bad ones, the overall effect of the drugs is good. Others of these drugs antagonize the chemical system inside the cell, such as the purine system or the folate system. From the patient's standpoint, it doesn't really make too much difference how they work.

The major short-term worry with these drugs is that they can destroy bone-marrow cells. The bone-marrow cells make red cells that carry oxygen, white cells that fight infection, and platelets that stop bleeding. Any of these blood-cell types can be suppressed by taking enough of these drugs, and even if there seem to be enough white cells, dangerous infections can occur.

These infections are often called "opportunistic," which means that they are caused by different kinds of germs than those that cause infections in healthy people. For example, patients are often afflicted with herpes zoster (shingles) and can be prone to infections from types of fungi that are around all the time but seldom cause disease. Or a rare bacterial infection can occur. These infections can be difficult to treat and sometimes hard to diagnose.

For patients who have taken immunosuppressant drugs for several years, there is some concern about cancer. Although this seems to be extremely rare or absent in humans, these drugs do cause cancer in some laboratory animals. It seems that if humans are afflicted, it is only after years of treatment. Present evidence suggests that leukemia can occasionally be caused by cytotoxic drugs such as cyclophosphamide, but not by methotrexate or azathioprine.

After considering all these dangers, we really don't know how to compare immunosuppressant drugs to other drugs. Although there is some potential danger of cancer, the alternative might be prednisone with all of its potential problems. It is possible that these drugs are actually less dangerous than some of the drugs with which we feel more comfortable.

In Wegener's granulomatosis, previously fatal, these drugs are usually curative. They are very helpful in severe polyarteritis. They are probably useful in resistant severe dermatomyositis or polymyositis. They are probably helpful in severe kidney disease of systemic lupus. They are very helpful and increasingly used in psoriatic arthritis and rheumatoid arthritis.

Methotrexate

2.5 mg round yellow tablet

Purpose: For reduction of inflammation and to retard disease progression.

Indications: Rheumatoid arthritis, dermatomyositis or polymyositis, psoriatic arthritis, other forms of synovitis.

Dosage: If taken orally, as is usual in rheumatoid arthritis, the dose is usually 5 to 15 mg per week given in two or three doses, twelve hours apart, sometimes as a single weekly dose. It should not be taken every day.

Side effects: These include opportunistic infections, mouth ulcers, and stomach problems. Damage to the liver, a special side effect of this drug, is particularly a problem if the drug is taken orally every day. When taken orally, this drug is absorbed by the intestine and passes through the liver on the way to general circulation. As a result, most doctors have discontinued this daily method of administration. Instead the drug is given intermittently, once a week, so that the liver has an opportunity to heal. Problems can still occur with the newer dose schedules, but are much less frequent. A severe problem with the lungs is occasionally seen with methotrexate. Cancer has not been reported.

Liver Function Tests

Methotrexate can, in rare cases, damage the liver: Enzymes can leak out of damaged liver cells and this can be measured in the blood. Liver function tests are used to detect damage before it becomes severe. The tests include bilirubin (jaundice), serum albumin, and serum alkaline phosphatase. The most important, however, are the liver enzymes SGOT (also called AST or ASAT) and SGPT (also called ALT or ALAT). Usually, test values should be below 40. With methotrexate therapy, they are usually measured every four to eight weeks, at least for the first one or two years, and then if normal perhaps less often. If they are abnormal more than one-half of the time it can be a signal to reduce dose or to consider a liver biopsy.

Special hints: This drug is extremely effective in many cases of rheumatoid arthritis and has become the preferred drug for many patients. Because of its remarkable effectiveness, it is now the most frequently used of the DMARDs. Regular blood tests are required, as with all of these drugs. Some doctors recommend liver biopsy to be sure that the liver is normal before starting the drug. However, this procedure is hazardous and is not necessary as long as blood liver tests are normal before the drug is started. A "baseline" liver biopsy is no longer recommended unless the patient already has a liver problem, in which case the drug probably should not be used anyway. Since alcohol also can damage the liver, alcohol intake should be extremely moderate during this period of methotrexate treatment. Some doctors recommend liver biopsy after a few years of treatment to make sure that no scarring has occurred. Current belief is that this is not necessary unless the liver blood tests are consistently abnormal. At this time, there seem to be worse complications from liver biopsies (the death rate is between one in a thousand and one in ten thousand) than from methotrexate liver disease (only about 40 serious events reported yet). Patients who are taking Plaquenil together with methotrexate seem to have fewer liver-test abnormalities.

Imuran (azathioprine), 6-MP (6-mercaptopurine)

50 mg scored, hourglass-shaped yellow to off-white tablet

Purpose: For immunosuppression.

Indications: Severe systemic lupus erythematosus, rheumatoid arthritis, psoriatic arthritis, steroid-resistant polymyositis or dermatomyositis.

Dosage: 100 to 150 mg (two or three tablets) daily is the usual dose.

Side effects: Azathioprine and 6-mercaptopurine are closely related drugs with almost identical actions. Azathioprine is the more frequently used. Side effects include opportunistic infections and possibility of late development of cancer, so far rare to absent in humans. Gastrointestinal (stomach) distress is occasionally noted. Hair loss is unusual, and there appears to be little effect on the sperm or the eggs. There are no bladder problems. Although liver damage has been reported, the drug is usually well tolerated.

Special hints: Regular blood tests are required. Patients taking Imuran or 6-MP should never take allopurinol (Zyloprim, a drug used to treat gout) at the same time since the combination of drugs can be fatal.

Once the patient responds to Imuran or 6-MP, it is often possible to reduce the dose. Theoretically, this decreases the risk of late side effects. Azathioprine has been shown to slow down the progression of rheumatoid arthritis and is very effective in some patients. Most people seem not to have any side effects but there is still concern about what might happen over the long run.

Sandimmune (cyclosporine)

25 mg capsules

100 mg capsules

Purpose: To reduce inflammation and disease progression in rheumatoid arthritis.

Indications: For reduction of inflammation in difficult severe rheumatoid arthritis not responsive to other agents. (Not an approved use by the Food and Drug Administration.)

Dosage: Use in rheumatoid arthritis is generally 3–5 mg per kilogram body weight per day. For a 150-pound (70 kg) person, this is 250 to 350 mg per day.

Side effects: The principal adverse reactions are kidney failure, tremor, excess hair growth, and problems with the gums. In rheumatoid arthritis the major problem has been with the kidneys, and this often requires discontinuation of the drug. The kidney failure is generally reversible.

Special hints: Cyclosporine was developed as a drug to prevent rejection of kidney, heart, and other organ transplants. It is a strong immunosuppressant. In rheumatoid arthritis its use is reserved for severely affected persons and it should be given only by physicians who are thoroughly familiar with its use. It can be very effective in some patients. The problem in rheumatoid arthritis patients is the kidney damage and this occurs at lower doses than in transplant patients. Hence, the dose is lower for rheumatoid arthritis patients. Some patients have had severe disease flare-ups after stopping cyclosporine. Researchers are exploring several ways to reduce the kidney problems, and there may be some progress in this area soon.

DRUGS TO REDUCE PAIN

This section is included mainly to emphasize that pain-reducing drugs except plain acetaminophen (Tylenol) have little place in the treatment of arthritis. Consider their four major disadvantages. First, they don't do anything for the arthritis; they just cover it up. Second, they help defeat the pain mechanism that tells you when you are doing something that is injuring your body. If you suppress it, you may injure your body without being aware of it. Third, the body adjusts to pain medicines, so that they aren't very effective over the long term. This phenomenon is called *tolerance* and develops to some extent with all of the drugs we commonly use. Fourth, pain medicines can have major side effects. The side effects range from stomach distress to constipation to mental changes. Most of these drugs are "downers," which you don't need if you have arthritis. You need to be able to cope with a somewhat more diffi-cult living situation than the average person. These drugs decrease your ability to solve problems.

Many individuals develop a tragic dependence on these agents. In arthri-tis, the addiction is somewhat different from what we usually imagine. Most people with arthritis are not truly physically addicted to codeine or Percodan or Demerol. They are psychologically dependent on these drugs as a crutch and become inordinately concerned with an attempt to eliminate every last symptom as a pretext for continuing medication. These agents conflict with the attempt to achieve independent living.

By and large, use these drugs only for the short term and only when rest-ing the sore part, so that you don't reinjure it while the pain is suppressed. Drugs mentioned first in this list are less harmful than those listed later. Drugs to reduce inflammation, discussed above, may reduce pain through direct pain action as well as through reduction of inflammation. This is preferable in inflammatory arthritis. In osteoarthritis, a plain acetaminophen (Tylenol, other brands) is often very useful as a nontoxic pain reliever.

These same principles hold for a number of less common pain relievers not described in the following section.

acetaminophen (Tylenol, percogesic)

325 mg white tablet or caplet
500 mg white tablet or caplet
500 mg yellow-and-red gel capsule

Purpose: For temporary relief of minor pain.

Indications: Mild temporary pain, particularly with cartilage degeneration (osteoarthritis).

Dosage: Two tablets (600-650 mg) every four hours as needed.

Side effects: Minimal. Unlike aspirin, acetaminophen usually does not upset the stomach, does not cause ringing in the ears, does not affect the clotting of the blood, does not interact with other medications, and is about as safe as can be. Of course, as with any drug, there are occasional problems, but this drug is frequently recommended in place of aspirin for children because of its greater safety. Acetaminophen is the only drug in this category that is not addictive. Overdose can result in severe liver damage.

Special hints: Acetaminophen is not anti-inflammatory; thus it is not an aspirin substitute in the treatment of arthritis. If the condition is a noninflammatory one such as osteoarthrosis, then it may be approximately as useful as aspirin with fewer side effects. It is only a mild pain reliever and therefore has fewer disadvantages than the following agents. It is relatively inexpensive. More heavily advertised names, such as Tylenol, may be more expensive than other acetaminophens. You need to read the labels. Consider the store brands.

Darvon (darvon compound, darvotran, darvocet, darvocet-N, propoxyphene)

Darvon: 32 mg, 65 mg pink capsule
darvon compound: 32 mg gray-and-pink capsule; 65 mg gray-and-red capsule
Darvocet-N: 50 mg, 100 mg coated, capsule-shaped dark-orange tablets

Purpose: Mild pain relief.

Indications: For short-term use in decreasing mild pain.

Dosage: One half grain (32 mg) or one grain (65 mg) every four hours as needed for pain.

Side effects: These drugs are widely promoted and have been widely used with a reasonably good safety record. In some cases, side effects may be due to use of aspirin or other medication in combination with the Darvon. Most worrisome to us has been the mentally dull feeling that many individuals report, sometimes described as a gray semi-unhappy fog. Others do not seem to notice this effect. Side reactions include dizziness, headache, sedation, paradoxical excitement, skin rash, and gastrointestinal disturbances.

Special hints: Darvon is not anti-inflammatory and is thus not an aspirin substitute. The pain relief given is approximately equal to that of aspirin in most cases. The drug is more expensive than aspirin or acetaminophen. It can induce dependence, particularly after long-term use.

Codeine (Empirin #3, 4; Tylenol #1, 2, 3, 4; aspirin with codeine #2, 3, 4; Vicodin)

Codeine (Empirin): 30 mg, 60 mg codeine round white tablet
Tylenol: 8 mg, 15 mg, 30 mg, 60 mg codeine round white tablet
Vicodin: 5 mg, 500 mg capsule-shaped white tablet

Purpose: Moderate pain relief.

Indications: For moderate pain relief over the short term.

Dosage: For some curious reason, the strength of codeine is often coded by number. For example, Empirin with codeine #1 or just Empirin #1 contains one eighth grain or 8 mg of codeine per tablet; #2 contains one fourth grain or 16 mg; #3 contains one half grain or 32 mg; and #4 contains one grain or 65 mg of codeine phosphate. A common dosage is a #3 tablet (32 mg codeine) every four hours as needed for pain.

Side effects: The side effects are proportional to the dosage. The more you take, the more side effects you are likely to have. Allergic reactions are quite rare.

Codeine is a narcotic. Thus, it can lead to addiction, with tolerance and drug dependence. Frequently in persons with arthritis it leads to constipation and sometimes a set of complications including fecal impaction and diverticulitis. More worrisome is the way that persons using codeine seem to lose their will to cope. The person taking codeine for many years sometimes seems sluggish and generally depressed. We don't really know whether the codeine is responsible, but we do think that codeine often makes it more difficult for the person with arthritis to cope with the very real problems that abound. The older patient can develop substantial complications from constipation caused by the codeine.

Percodan (Percobarb, Percodan-Demi, Percogesic)

Percodan: yellow tablets
Percodan-Demi: pink tablets

Purpose: For pain relief.

Indications: For short-term relief of moderate to severe pain.

Dosage: One tablet every six hours as needed.

Side effects: Percodan is a curious combination drug. The basic narcotic is oxycodone, to which is added aspirin and other minor pain relievers. Combination drugs have a number of theoretical disadvantages, but Percodan is a strong and effective reliever of pain. It does require a special prescription because it is a strong narcotic and the hazards of serious addiction are present. The manufacturers state that the habit-forming potentialities are somewhat less than with morphine and somewhat greater than with codeine. The drug is usually well tolerated.

Special hints: Percodan is a good drug for people with cancer, but it is very dangerous in the treatment of arthritis. It is not an anti-inflammatory agent and does not work directly on any of the disease processes. It is habit forming and it does break the pain reflex. It is a mental depressant, and can result in serious addiction.

Demerol (meperidine)

Demerol-Hydrochloride: 50 mg, 100 mg scored, round white tablets
Demerol APAP: 50 mg pink-and-dark pink splotches

Purpose: For relief of severe pain such as in cancer, heart attacks, kidney stones.

Indications: For temporary relief of severe pain, as with a bad fracture that has been immobilized.

Dosage: Various preparations are available that contain 25 mg, 50 mg, or 100 mg of Demerol. One tablet every four hours for pain is a typical dose. Dose is increased for more severe pain and decreased for milder pain.

Side effects: Demerol is a major narcotic approximately equivalent to morphine in pain relief capacity and in addiction potential. Tolerance develops and increasing doses may be required. Drug dependence and severe withdrawal symptoms may be seen if the drug is stopped. Psychological dependence also occurs. The underlying disease may be covered up and serious symptoms may be masked. Nausea, vomiting, constipation, and a variety of other side effects may occur.

Special hints: This is not a drug for the treatment of arthritis. Stay away from it.

TRANQUILIZERS

Valium, Librium, and other tranquilizers are among the most prescribed drugs in North America. They do not help arthritis. These drugs depress the patient and should be avoided by persons with arthritis whenever possible.

MUSCLE RELAXANTS

Soma, Flexeril, and a number of other agents are prescribed frequently as "muscle relaxants." In general, these act like tranquilizers. They treat only symptoms, and are usually not helpful in arthritis. One exception: Flexeril is sometimes useful against fibromyalgia.

ANTIDEPRESSANTS

There is a role for antidepressant treatment in arthritis when depression is a problem, and in selected cases it can be helpful. More frequently, a low dose of an antidepressant such as Elavil is given at bedtime, not to fight depression but to help improve the quality of sleep and to reduce the problems of fibromyalgia.

NAMES AND AVAILABILITIES

Some drugs are known by different names in the United States, Canada, New Zealand, and Australia. In addition, because of drugs' differing status in terms of government approval, some drugs available in one country are not available in another. All prescription drugs must be taken under the direction of a medical doctor, however, so follow your doctor's guidelines on what to use.

The chart on the following pages includes drugs approved for arthritis treatment in the U.S. It does not include medications approved in other countries but not in the U.S. For information about any drug whose name does not appear in this chart, speak to your doctor or pharmacist.

INTERNATIONAL AVAILABILITY OF DRUGS

UNITED STATES	CANADA	UNITED KINGDOM	AUSTRALIA	NEW ZEALAND	SOUTH AFRICA
(acetylsalicylic acid)* aspirin* Ecotrin*	Novasen Aspirin Arthrinol Arthrin Ecotrin Entrophen	aspirin Benoral (benorylate: aspirin-paracetamol esther)	aspirin Dispersible Alkaseltzer ASA Aspro Ecotrin Winsprin	aspirin Disprin Aspec 300 Aspro Tab Cortia Tab Ecotrin Solprin	aspirin Aspasol Compral Disprin Aspro Suparin
Disalcid (salsalate)	Disalciol	Disalcid (salsalate)	not available	not available	not available
Trilisate (choline magnesium trisalicylate)	Trilisate	not available	not available	not available	not available
Nuprin* Advil* (ibuprofen)	Amersol (APO-ibuprofen) Nuprin Advil Actiprofen Medipren	Brufen Junifen sugar-free syrup Brufen Retard Fenbid (ibuprofen) codafen continus (ibuprofen + codeine)	ibuprofen Brufen	Brufen Nurofen Anafen Pamored Panafen	Nurofen Antifam Adco-ibuprofen Brufen Betaprofen Inza
Ansaid (flurbiprofen)	Ansaid Froben	Froben Froben SR (flurbiprofen)	not available	Froben	Froben

Generic drugs are listed in parentheses. Those marked with an asterisk are available without a prescription.

INTERNATIONAL AVAILABILITY OF DRUGS (continued)

UNITED STATES	CANADA	UNITED KINGDOM	AUSTRALIA	NEW ZEALAND	SOUTH AFRICA
Clinoril (sulindac)	Clinoril (APO-sulin) Novo Sudac	Clinoril (Sulindac)	Aclin Clinoril	Clinoril Sulindac	Clinoril
Daypro (oxaprozin)	Daypro	not available	not available	not available	not available
Dolobid (Diflunisal)	Dolobid	Dolobid	Dolobid	Dolobid Diflunisal Ansal	Diflunisal
Feldene (piroxicam)	Feldene (APO-piroxicam) Novo-Pirecam	Feldene	Feldene	Feldene Piroxicam APO-Proxicam Candyl-D Piram	Feldene
Indocin (indomethacin)	Indocid Novo-Methacin APO-Indomethacin	Indomethacin Indocid Indocid R Imbrilon Indomax SR Rheumacin SR Indomod Indolar SR Flexin continus	Indocid	Indocid Indomethacin Arthrexin Rheumacin	Arthrexan Articulen Betacin Indocid Indomed Methabid
Lodine (etodolac)	not available	Lodine Lodine SR (etodolac)	not available	not available	not available

INTERNATIONAL AVAILABILITY OF DRUGS *(continued)*

UNITED STATES	CANADA	UNITED KINGDOM	AUSTRALIA	NEW ZEALAND	SOUTH AFRICA
Meclomen (meclofenamate)	Mefenamic Acid (ponslan)	Mefenamic Acid Ponstan Dysman Ponstan forte	not available	Ponslan Mefanamicaid Mefic	not available
Motrin Rufen (ibuprofen)	ibuprofen Motrin APO-ibuprofen Novo-Profen	Motrin Nurofen	Rafen	Brufen ibuprofen Anafen Nurofen Panored Panafen	Antiflam Betaprofen Brufen Inza Nurofen
Nalfon (fenoprofen)	Nalfon	Fenopron Progesic (fenoprofen)	not available	discontinued	Fenoprofen
Naprosyn Aleve* (naproxen)	Naprosyn (APO-naproxen) Naxen Anaprox Novo-Naprox	Naproxen Naprosyn SR Nycopren Synflex Pranoxen continus Napratec (naproxen + misoprostol)	Naprosyn Naprogesic Naprosyn SR Inza	Naprosyn APO-Naproxen Naxen Nofian Naprogesic	Naprosyn Nafasol Naxen Synflex

Generic drugs are listed in parentheses. Those marked with an asterisk are available without a prescription.

INTERNATIONAL AVAILABILITY OF DRUGS (continued)

UNITED STATES	CANADA	UNITED KINGDOM	AUSTRALIA	NEW ZEALAND	SOUTH AFRICA
Orudis Oruvail (ketoprofen)	Novo-Profen Orudis Oruvail Rhodis APO-Keto-E	Orudis* Oruvail (ketoprofen) Alrheumat	Orudis Orudis SR Oruvail	Oruvail Ketoprofen Kapren Kefen Orudis	Oruvail
Relafen (nabumetone)	Relafen (nabumetone)	Relifex (nabumetone)	not available	Relafen	Relifen
Tolectin (tolmetin sodium)	Tolectin	Tolmetin Tolectin	not available	not available	Tolmetin
Toradol (ketorolac)	Toradol (ketorolac)	Toradol (ketorolac- trometamol)	Torodol	not available	not available
Voltaren Cataflam (diclofenac)	Voltaren SR Voltaren Novo-Difenac APO-Diclo	Voltarol (R) Diclofenac sodium Diclomax Retard Arthrotec (diclofenac + misoprostal)	Voltaren Fenac	Voltaren Diclofenac APO-Diclofenac Anfenax SR Diclax	Arcanafenac Cliniflam Difenac Flexagen Panamor Voltaren
Prednisone (oral steroid)	Prednisone Deltasone APO-Prednisone Novo-Prednisone Winpred	Prednisolone	Prednisone Prednisolone	APO-Prednisone	Prednisolone Meticortelone Predeltilone Pred-Forte Pred-Mild Predsol

INTERNATIONAL AVAILABILITY OF DRUGS (continued)

UNITED STATES	CANADA	UNITED KINGDOM	AUSTRALIA	NEW ZEALAND	SOUTH AFRICA
Depo-Medrol (injectable steroid)	Depo-Medrol	Dexamethasone Decadron Hydrocortistab (hydrocortisone acetate) Depo-medrone (prednisolone acetate) Adcortyl Kenolog Lederspan (triamcinolone hexacetonide)	Depo-Medrol	Depo-Medrol	Depo-Medrol
Myochrysine Solganol (injectable gold salts)	Myochrisine Solganol	Myocrisine (injectable sodium aurothiamalate)	Gold 50 Myocrisine	Myocrisine Sodium Aurothiomalate	Myocrisine
Ridaura (auranofin)	Ridaura Aurandfin	Ridaura Auranofin (oral gold salts)	Ridaura Auranofin	Ridaura Auranofin	Ridaura
Penicillamine (cuprimine)	Cuprimine Depen	Penicillamine Distamine Pendramine	D-Penamine	D-Penicillamine D-Peramine	Penicillamine Metalcaptase

Generic drugs are listed in parentheses. Those marked with an asterisk are available without a prescription.

INTERNATIONAL AVAILABILITY OF DRUGS (continued)

UNITED STATES	CANADA	UNITED KINGDOM	AUSTRALIA	NEW ZEALAND	SOUTH AFRICA
Plaquenil (hydroxychloroquine)	Plaquenil (hydroxychloroquine)	Plaquenil	Plaquenil	Plaquenil Hydroxychloroquine	Chloroquin Nivaquine Hydroxychloroquine
Azulfidine (sulfasalazine)	Salazopyrin SAS Enteric-500 PMS-Sylfasalazine	Salazopyrin (EN) (sulphasalazine)	Salazopyrine En Tabs	Salazopyrin Sulphasalazine Colizine	Salazopyrin
Rheumatrex (methotrexate)	Methotrexate Rheumatrex Amethopterin	Methotrexate Matrex	Ledertrexate Methoblastin	Methotrexate Ledertrexate Methoblastin	Methotrexate
Imuran (azathioprine)	Imuran Azathioprine	Imuran (azathioprine)	Imuran	Imuran Azathioprine Thioprine	Azapress Imuran
Sandimmune (cyclosporine)		Sandimmune (cyclosporine) Cyclophosphamide Endoxana Leukeran (chlorambucil)	Sandimmune	Sandimmune Cyclosporin	Sandimmune
(acetaminophen)* (paracetamol) Tylenol*	acetaminophen Tylenol Atasol Exdol Panadol Rounox	not available Paracetamol Co-codamol Kapake Solpadol Tylex (Paracetamol + codeine) Remedeine (Paracetamol + dihydrocodeine) Co-proxamol (Paracetamol + dextropropoxyphene) Fortagesic (Paracetamol + Pentazocine) Lobak (Paracetamol + chlormezanone)	Panadol Panamax Dymadon Tylenol (Paracetamol + codeine)	APO-Paracetamol Panadol Dispinol Panol Paraspen Paratabs	(Paracetamol) Calpol Dolorol Ennagesic Panado Pyragesic

INTERNATIONAL AVAILABILITY OF DRUGS (continued)

UNITED STATES	CANADA	UNITED KINGDOM	AUSTRALIA	NEW ZEALAND	SOUTH AFRICA
Darvon (propoxyphene)	Darvon Prosst's 642's	not available	Digesic	Digesic (Paracetamol & propoxyphen)	Doloxene Distalgesic
codeine	codeine Phosphate	codeine	codeine	codeine Paracetamol	codeine
Percodan (percobarb percogesic)	Percodan-Demi Percodan	not available	Codalgin Codral Dymadon Co Panadeine	not available	not available
Percocet	Percocet Oxycocet Endococet	not available	Panamax Co Paracetamol & codeine		
Demerol (meperidine)	Demerol	not available	Codis Aspalgin Codiphen Disprin Forte Solcode Aspirin & codeine	Pethidine	not available

Generic drugs are listed in parentheses. Those marked with an asterisk are available without a prescription.

▼ ▼ ▼ ▼ ▼ ▼ ▼

21. What About Surgery?

Surgery can relieve pain, restore function, and return a patient to employ-ment. Its potential to satisfactorily repair a damaged joint increases year by year. But surgery is expensive and painful, is associated with a long recovery period, keeps you away from activities during the period of convalescence, and may not be successful. The joint might be worse after-ward. Surgery can even kill you or paralyze you, although this is rare. The decision to undergo surgery is one that you will make with your doctor. It's a major step and you want to make the right decision. Here are some guidelines to help you sort out the issues.

GENERAL RULES

Surgery for Arthritis Is Seldom Urgent

With only a few exceptions, a delay of days, weeks, or even months makes relatively little difference with surgery for arthritis. If the operation is successful, you will still have the good results to enjoy; if the operation is unsuccessful, you will have delayed the pain and expense by waiting. You have plenty of time for a second opinion, or a third. You can watch your condition to see if it will go away by itself or perhaps stabilize at an acceptable level. So take your time. Rare exceptions to this rule include bone conditions causing nerve pressure, a bacterial infection in the bone or joint, or a rupture of the tendons.

Not All Surgeons Are Equal

Generally, you will want an orthopedic or hand surgeon to perform any oper-ations on your joints that may be required. You will also want a surgeon who does a lot of joint operations and is up-to-date on the latest techniques. Surgery is a rapidly changing field, and familiarity with the most recent advances leads to better results. A surgeon who performs the operation only once or twice a year is not likely to have the same level of skill as a surgeon who does the operation weekly. As a dividend, you will usually find that the busy joint surgeon is more conservative in his or her recommendation for operation. It's not at all uncommon for a good orthopedic surgeon to indicate quite candidly that the condition for which the operation is being considered is not likely to respond to surgical treatment—and then you will be spared an unsuccessful operation.

Not All Operations Are Equal

The total hip replacement and total knee replacement are very fine operations—almost all patients receive some benefit from them. On the other hand, certain procedures, such as tendon operations on the small joints of the hand or most kinds of back surgery, are far less predictable. Before you decide to have either of the latter two kinds of operation, you will want to find out how good the recommended operation is.

Best Results Are Achieved When Problems Are Localized

Medical treatment is often best for a widespread problem. On the other hand, if the problem is localized, say in one knee, then surgery is likely to be a good, targeted approach to the problem. If a large number of joints are involved, surgery may be impractical. For example, the lower extremity has eight major weight-bearing areas: the two forefeet, the ankles, the knees, and the hips. If any one of these areas is limiting walking, surgery may be a wise move. But if all eight areas are bad, then fixing one is not going to be of particular help. Improvement in one joint without relief to the other seven cannot be translated into function and increased activity. Be realistic. Ask how well you would be if the area of a proposed operation were entirely well. If the answer is, "It wouldn't be much different," then surgery may not be advisable.

Best Results Are Achieved in Treatment of Large Joints

The joint is a complicated structure, and healing after surgery can result in stiffness, particularly if the surface area of the joint is small. The best surgical procedures repair large joints such as the hip and the knee. Results in these areas are usually predictably good. With the smaller joints, sophisticated repair techniques sometimes don't improve function significantly and should be approached with caution. Usually problems with smaller joints are also problems that involve many joints, which again complicates the surgical approach.

SPECIFIC OPERATIONS

Joint Replacement

This is the newest and by far the most important orthopedic surgical procedure for arthritis. The joint is removed and replaced entirely by an artificial joint. The cartilage is replaced by long-wearing plastics such as Teflon, the bone is replaced by stainless steel, and the artificial joint is embedded in the ends of the bones on either side by a marvelous cement called methyl methacralate. This bone cement made the new era in joint surgery possible by providing a way to anchor the artificial joint to the bones.

The hip was the first joint to be replaced. Total hip replacement is an excellent operation in the hands of an experienced surgeon. Pain is almost totally relieved and function is greatly improved. The present artificial hip is estimated to last ten to fifteen years, and newer models are expected to last longer as design problems are overcome. The failure rate is only one or two percent, but these patients may have infections or even have to have the artificial hip removed. It is true that some patients receiving artificial hips have had to have a replacement for the replacement; it is also true that this usually has been satisfactory. Recently, a new type of total hip operation has been developed that works by allowing bony ingrowth into the artificial joint and that does not require cement.

The knee is a complicated hinge joint with a requirement for sideways stability. This has made it more difficult to construct an appropriate replacement joint, since the joint must move freely in the hinge direction but must strongly resist sideways force. The ball-and-socket joint of the hip poses easier engineering problems. Techniques of knee replacement have been greatly refined over the last several years.

Ankle replacements remain less frequently used. Shoulder replacements have become quite good. Operations to replace the small joints of the fingers are widely practiced, but the outcome has not been uniformly satisfactory. One of the problems with present operations for the small joints of the hands is that appearance may be considerably improved by the straightening of deformed fingers, but the ability to use the hand may not be greatly changed.

Synovectomy

Removal of inflamed synovium is termed a synovectomy. This popular operation results in a reduction of the swelling of synovitis and presumably less enzymatic damage to the joint because the inflamed tissue mass has been reduced. Unfortunately, joint stiffness is often experienced after the synovectomy and the inflamed tissue frequently grows back. There has been a long-standing argument about whether synovectomy should be done early or late (or never) in rheumatoid arthritis, with some doctors holding each extreme position. In other words, the effects of synovectomy are not so dramatic that people can't argue about them. There should be a special reason for this operation, such as worsening of a single joint when all other joints are in control or the hope of avoiding the use of a hazardous drug.

Resections

Some older operations sound a bit strange, and this is the case with resection procedures. Here, bones are just cut away and removed. This sounds as though it wouldn't be very helpful, but it often is. Resection of the metatarsal heads in the forefoot, for example, can relieve pain and restore the ability to walk. Similar operations may be done in the distal ulna, the bone on the outside of the wrist. Bunions and other protuberances can be removed. While this type of surgery is not elegant in concept, it can be very useful.

Fusions

An operation to unite two bones is termed a *fusion*. Such operations are useful to stabilize joints; the fusion provides a platform for movement and prevents pain in the fused area. The wrist and ankle are the joints where this procedure is most frequently used; fusion of the back or part of the neck is also performed on occasion. A successful fusion, limiting all motion, stops pain. In the area that is fused, flexibility is lost. Usually a fusion places additional strain on nearby joints that are called on to take over the flexibility functions. Fusion doesn't always work, and nonunion can occur. These operations are useful, however, in certain situations.

Back Surgery

A full discussion about indications for back surgery is beyond the scope of this chapter. Most patients know from talking with friends that unsuccessful back surgery is common. In most cases, the doctor was not very enthusiastic about performing this surgery but the continuing problems of the patient eventually led doctor and patient to agree on this measure. And it didn't work.

By and large, back surgery is not advisable unless there is evidence of pressure on nerve roots. This may happen with a herniated disk, or with narrowing of the spinal canal, or with back fractures.

Myelography is a special X-ray technique for obtaining an X-ray image of the spinal cord. A myelogram can demonstrate pressure on the nerves in the spinal cord. Operations in patients with negative myelograms are the least likely to succeed. However, the myelogram itself requires placement of a needle into the spinal canal and the injection of a not-innocuous dye into the space around the spinal cord. It is uncomfortable, and there are some side effects. Hence, even considering a myelogram should be reserved for the most serious back problems. Now a CT scan can provide much of the same information. The CT scan involves some radiation and is expensive, but generally safe. It doesn't hurt. The newer magnetic resonance (MR) imaging tests don't involve radiation. They are expensive, but they can be very helpful.

The back is composed of an extraordinarily complex set of muscles, ligaments, and tendons. The injury may be anywhere and is frequently not in the spine; hence, surgery on the spine may not be countering what is wrong. Seek multiple opinions before having a back operation. You want to avoid back surgery if you can, and it's mainly up to you.

Neurological Operations

There can be pressure on nerves out in the limbs. An example is the carpal tunnel syndrome, where there is pressure on the nerve passing over the front of the wrist resulting in pain and tingling in the fingers. This pressure can be effectively eliminated by surgery and surgery should be considered if rest and/or injection do not result in disappearance of the syndrome within a few weeks. Other problems, such as a Morton's neuroma, can also cause peripheral pain. Here, an injury has caused the nerve fibers to grow into a little ball and to transmit pain signals all the time. If this bundle of nerves is removed, the pain is eliminated and a good result obtained. So while we can't really operate to repair nerves, we can either remove the structures that are pressing on them or remove the area that is sending the abnormal signals.

"Cosmetic" Surgery

Usually, surgery for a joint should be done only to relieve pain or to improve function. The appearance of the joint is much less important. Some operations serve mainly to improve appearance. Many patients are later disappointed by such operations. The appearance is less than perfect anyway, and the patient somehow has been expecting that the part would work better if it looked better, despite advice to the contrary.

▼ ▼ ▼ ▼ ▼ ▼ ▼

Appendix: The Arthritis Foundation and the Arthritis Society—International Locations

THE ARTHRITIS Foundation in the United States, New Zealand, and Australia and the Arthritis Society in Canada are truly marvelous institutions. They sponsor programs in public education and professional education, support young professionals establishing research careers in arthritis, and provide direct support for research activities. They lead the fight for increased government programs of research and service.

The Arthritis Foundation or Society consists of a national office and local chapters or branches around the country. You will usually want to contact the local chapter, which can advise you of doctors and clinics in your area, provide instructional materials, and occasionally help with financial problems. There may be a schedule of activities you could attend. Or you might want to volunteer your efforts.

Look in the telephone directory under the Arthritis Foundation or call 1-800-283-7800 for toll-free information. The address of the national office is:

UNITED STATES
The Arthritis Foundation
1314 Spring St., N.W.
Atlanta, GA 30309

GREAT BRITAIN
Arthritis Care
18 Stephenson Way
London, England NW1 2HD
Telephone (071) 916-1500

CANADA

The Arthritis Society
National Office
250 Bloor St. East, Suite 901
Toronto, Ontario M4W 3P2
Telephone: (416) 967-1414

The Arthritis Society
Newfoundland Division
P.O. Box 522, Station C
St. John's, Newfoundland A1C 5K4
Telephone: (709) 368-8190

The Arthritis Society
Prince Edward Island Division
P.O. Box 4116
Bedeque, P.E.I. C0B 1C0
Telephone: (902) 887-3524
    or 1-800-565-2873 (toll free)

The Arthritis Society
Nova Scotia Division
5516 Spring Garden Road
Halifax, Nova Scotia B3J 1G6
Telephone: (902) 429-7025
    or 1-800-565-2873 (toll free)

The Arthritis Society
New Brunswick Division
65 Brunswick Street
Fredericton, New Brunswick E3B 1G5
Telephone: (506) 457-1652

The Arthritis Society
Quebec Division
2155 Guy Street, Suite 1120
Montreal, Quebec H3H 2R9
Telephone: (514) 846-8840
    or 1-800-335-6175 (toll free)

The Arthritis Society
Ontario Division
250 Bloor Street East, Suite 901
Toronto, Ontario M4W 3P2
Telephone: (416) 967-1414
    or 1-800-361-1112 (toll free)

The Arthritis Society
Manitoba Division
386 Broadway, Suite 105
Winnipeg, Manitoba R3C 3R6
Telephone: (204) 942-4892

The Arthritis Society
Saskatchewan Division
2078 Halifax Street
Regina, Saskatchewan S4P 1T7
Telephone: (306) 352-3312
    or 1-800-667-0097 (toll free)

The Arthritis Society
Alberta & N.W.T. Division
105, 1301 – 8th Street S.W.
Calgary, Alberta T2R 1B7
Telephone: (403) 228-2571
    or 1-800-332-1316 (toll free)

The Arthritis Society
British Columbia & Yukon Division
895 West 10th Avenue
Vancouver, British Columbia V5Z 1L7
Telephone: (604) 871-4537
    or 1-800-667-2847 (toll free)

SOUTH AFRICA
Arthritis Foundation of South Africa
Head Office
709 Tulbagh Center
Capetown, 8001
South Africa

AUSTRALIA

Arthritis Foundation of the
    Australian Capital Territory
G.P.O. Box 1642
Canberra City, ACT 2601
Telephone: (06) 257-4842

AFA Australian Capital Territory
P.O. Box 352
Woden, ACT 2606
Telephone: (062) 81-6814

Arthritis Foundation of Australia
National Office
P.O. Box 121
Sydney, NSW 2001
Telephone: (02) 221-2456

AFA New South Wales
P.O. Box 370
Darlinghurst, NSW 2010
Telephone: (02) 281-1611

Arthritis Foundation of
Queensland
P.O. Box 6060
Acacia Ridge 4110
Brisbane, Queensland
Telephone: (07) 274-1360

AFA South Australia
99 Anzac Highway
Ashford, SA 5035
Telephone: (08) 297-2488

Arthritis Foundation of Victoria
263-265 Kooyong Rd.
Elsternwick, Victoria 3185
Telephone: (03) 530-0255
P.O. Box 130
Caulfield
South 3162

Arthritis Foundation of Tasmania
P.O. Box 80
Burnie 7320
Tasmania

Western Australia Arthritis &
    Rheumatism Foundation
    (WAARF)
P.O. Box 34
Wembeley, WA 6014
Telephone: (09) 387-7066

Arthritis Foundation of the
Northern Territory
P.O. Box 37582
Winnellie 0821
Northern Territory

NEW ZEALAND

Arthritis Foundation of
    New Zealand
National Office
P.O. Box 10-020
Wellington
Telephone: (04) 721-427

Arthritis Foundation
Auckland Division
242 Great South Road
Green Lane
Auckland

Index

Page numbers in **boldface** indicate where you can find the most information on each topic.

ARTHRITIS: A Take Care of Yourself Health Guide for Arthritis

Fourth Edition

James F. Fries, M.D.

The Companion Volume to THE ARTHRITIS HELPBOOK
The Book that Answers All Your Questions About Arthritis

You can have much more control over your arthritis than you think. In this enormously helpful book, arthritis expert Dr. James Fries has created a program that will help you take an active role in understanding and defeating your arthritis. Fully revised to include the most up-to-date medical information, Dr. Fries' three-step program shows you how to

▼ Identify the kind of arthritis you have
▼ Work with a doctor to choose the best treatment and medication program
▼ Cope with the daily problems of pain

Thirty-one easy-to-read decision charts illustrate when to use home treatment and when to consult a doctor. There's also sensitive advice on dealing with emotional and sexual difficulties and a section that answers common questions about employment. With this book's wealth of information on all aspects of arthritis, no one who has arthritis can afford to be without it. Ask for ARTHRITIS by James Fries at your bookstore, or send the coupon below to:

> Addison-Wesley Publishing Company
> Retail Sales
> One Jacob Way
> Reading, MA 01867

Please send me _____ copy(ies) of ARTHRITIS: A TAKE CARE OF YOUR-SELF HEALTH GUIDE FOR ARTHRITIS @ $14.00 per copy.

My check or money order for full payment is enclosed. (Add state and local sales tax where applicable. Postage paid by Addison-Wesley.) Please allow four to six weeks for delivery.

Name _____

Address _____

City _____ State _____ Zip _____

Order Form
Audio Relaxation Cassettes

Send completed form to:
Stanford Arthritis Center
1000 Welch Rd., Suite 204
Palo Alto, CA 94304
Phone: (415) 723-7935

ITEM	HOW MANY

Time For Healing: Relaxation for Mind and Body
Designed to be used with the Arthritis Self-Management (Self-Help) Course, it includes two 30-minute relaxation exercises with background music and the voice of Catherine Regan, Ph.D.: *Progressive Muscle Relaxation* helps you achieve deep muscular relaxation and releases tension; it also quiets the mind and emotions. *Guided Imagery–A Walk in the Country* uses the imagination to travel to a pleasant place and time, helping you to achieve total relaxation and heightened self awareness. . . . . _____

Time for Healing: Shorter Version (Leader's Tape)
Designed to be used with the Arthritis Self-Management (Self-Help) Course, it includes condensed versions of the progressive muscle relaxation, and guided imagery exercises. . . . . _____

Total number of tapes ordered . . . . _____

PRICE: $8 each *(plus $.78 each for shipping, $1.85 for overseas shipping)*

BULK ORDERS: $6.00 each for orders of 10-24 *(plus $4 shipping, $20 for overseas shipping)*
$5.50 each for orders of 25-49 *(plus $6 shipping, $30 for overseas shipping)*
$5.00 each for orders of 50-99 *(shipping included)*
$4.50 each for orders of 100 or more *(shipping included)*

TOTAL . . . . $ _____

8.25% SALES TAX IN CALIFORNIA . . . . $ _____

SHIPPING . . . . $ _____

TOTAL ENCLOSED *(check made payable to*
CATHERINE A. REGAN, Ph.D.) . . . . $ _____

SHIP TO: _____

_____

_____

Time for Healing: Relaxation for Mind and Body (Spanish version)
same description and price as above *(make checks for this tape only* payable to Stanford University). . . . . _____

IMPORTANT NEWS
FOR PEOPLE WITH ARTHRITIS

Subscribe to *Arthritis Today* and get the most up-to-date information about living with arthritis. In addition to reviews of the latest medical research, you'll find news on dietary recommendations, financial planning strategies, exercise programs and special tips for traveling, as well as feature articles to give you insight on how to make life with arthritis more rewarding. Your annual $20 contribution also makes you a member of the Arthritis Foundation and helps fund vital research to find better treatments and cures for America's #1 crippling disease.

ARTHRITIS FOUNDATION®

*Your Source
for Help and Hope* ®

For instant membership
call toll-free in the U.S.

1-800-933-0032

MasterCard and VISA accepted.

Join now and receive a 7th issue FREE!

In addition to funding research, your membership helps local chapters of the Foundation around the country sponsor important programs including:

- Self-help education and training programs
- Supervised recreational exercise
- Information and referral services
- Clubs and support groups